Born Still

A Memoir of Grief

Janet Fraser

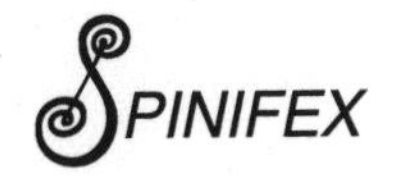

First published by Spinifex Press, 2020

Spinifex Press Pty Ltd
PO Box 5270, North Geelong, VIC 3215, Australia
PO Box 105, Mission Beach, QLD 4852, Australia

women@spinifexpress.com.au
www.spinifexpress.com.au

Edited by Pauline Hopkins, Renate Klein and Susan Hawthorne
Cover design by Deb Snibson, MAPG
Typesetting by Helen Christie, Blue Wren Books
Typeset in Minion Pro
Printed by McPherson's Printing Group

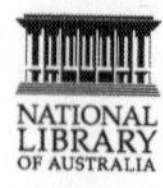

A catalogue record for this book is available from the National Library of Australia

ISBN: 9781925950120 (paperback)
ISBN: 9781925950137 (ebook: epub)

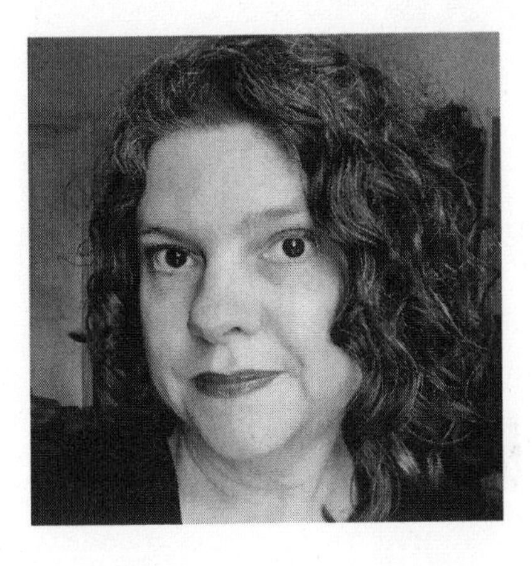

Janet Fraser is a mother, poet, historian and National Convenor of the Australian homebirth network, Joyous Birth. She writes about feminism, history, human rights, birth and parenting.

To C, I and R with love

Contents

Introduction

When Grief is Political

How many children do you have? An innocuous question, used thousands of times a day, as an entry into polite conversation. What you may not know is that sometimes when you ask that question of a stranger, they do a quick mental calculation before they answer. Are you likely to see them again? Are you in a position of authority over them? Do they feel like announcing a dead child in this interaction, or not? It's not always so simple. So this is the story of my answer and why I sometimes hesitate before I answer you.

This is a memoir but it is a very particular kind of memoir: it is a political memoir of grief. It is a deeply personal, viscerally revealing story that could only have occurred in a specific context. When feminists said the personal was political, they probably did not anticipate in how many ways we could use the concept. It is an idea which has helped save my life or at least my sanity since I know only too well how easy it is to become the next woman in the spotlight, the target, the witch's double. By placing my life in a political context it becomes easier to bear the weight of the hatred, betrayals and pain. The grief is another story but here too the political is personal. Or more precisely, the personal is political.

The Witch's Double: The Mother the System Tried to Crush

Around six thousand years ago, a young woman in what we now call Denmark, died along with her baby. Their community buried them in a joint grave. A flint knife indicating the baby's sex to be male was placed in the grave, and red beads were used to decorate the mother's hips. The baby was laid to rest on the outstretched wing of a swan. The poignancy of this scene speaks to us still because we recognise ourselves in this burial. Those of us who have experienced loss relate to the ritual of making a precious baby safe. Those of us touched by loss are moved by the deaths of both mother and baby. Despite our distance in time and our technology, the reality is that loss still occurs and can occur at any time throughout pregnancy and birth. I wonder though, would the Danish mourners recognise the current climate for loss?

The events I will describe took place between 2009 and 2012, and in a situation in Australian maternity politics that no longer exists because homebirth has been largely stamped out. Giving birth is now under obstetric control. I want to shed light on one argument used at that time to justify removing decision-making from Australian women: the trope of homebirthing women as a danger to our babies, to social cohesion, to ourselves and to other women.

It is a defining opportunity for me to have my own experience published in my own words after being ignored and sidelined for so long. During the events that unfolded, the media found it far easier to construct me as a witch than engage with my ideas. I always shy away from using 'witch craze' as a descriptor for this phenomenon of tearing women down in Australia. I discussed this with my friend, Petra Bueskens, recently, and she made the brilliant point that it is perhaps death in an online world which we experience rather than death at the stake. I have taken that to heart.

The current political context in which birth is becoming overtaken by gender neutral language – it is 'people' that give birth[1] – as if the embodied act of birthing could ever be separated from our biology – also brings a certain urgency to describing these experiences. We cannot spell out having a female body in a world in which hatred of women is a scourge, if we cannot say that women give birth. What happened to me was because of my female status and because of how I am therefore categorised as female in patriarchy. I will not separate my sexed body from those events that unfolded. As midwife Marylou Singleton puts it, "So essentially, we've taken this quintessential female process of gestating and giving birth, which is something biologically that female members of the species do, and we've erased all reference to people of the female sex."[2]

I also want to draw out the ways in which loss is described depending on the perceived level of social compliance of the woman, or girl, who is pregnant.

Briefly, I am the National Convenor of Joyous Birth, the Australian homebirth network. In 2009, I gave birth at home to my third child, Roisin. She was born still. From that moment, there was a deliberate calculation to smear me and undermine my capacity to resist both the medical establishment and the accepted understanding of what giving birth is all about. Everything from the ugly photos used by the media to the appointment of two women as Crown Solicitor and Counsel Assisting at the eventual inquest, was intended to warn other women: step out of line and beware the consequences. Strangely, no other woman in Australia has been through quite what I went through. Midwives are weeded out of their workplace via the coronial system, but mothers are usually used as witnesses in court to bring their midwives undone rather than be subject to scrutiny themselves. I am a mother the system tried to crush.

Two main pathologies were brought to bear on me when my stillbirth occurred. I was a mad, bad freebirther and, as I wrote after the inquest, "Freebirthers are the new whore: they are vicious, unregulated, uncaring, murderous, dangerous and probably hairy." I was further deemed by so-called medico-legal authorities, to have 'concealed' my pregnancy, a label with more than a hint of the 'madwoman in the attic' to it. One of the questions asked at the inquest was: "Does Janet Fraser pose a danger to public health?" So between my activism on behalf of birthing women and my refusal to be an obedient mother, public punishment had to be devised for me.

This book is about some of the experiences of my daughter's birth, the police investigation, the coronial inquiry and the personal aftermath over the last eight years since the inquest. There was a three-year wait from birth to inquest, which was a very long gestation. During that time I could not speak out. I've lost a decade of my life. I birthed Roisin at 40, then went into the underworld and emerged, blinking, in 2019 at 50. I am still chewing through the limb I've lost to the trap but perhaps bringing light to those years will speed the process. It certainly can't hurt.

This is not intended as an academic work, replete with footnotes and quotes. Any poetry is my own, unless otherwise stated. It is a reflection on my memory of these events and experiences. The pain of being called a liar over and over makes me very sensitive to cries that I am inventing what I'm writing. I am sure that were a person financially equipped, they could purchase the inquest transcription and produce a very different work. If I were approaching this as a historian, that's exactly what I'd hope to do. But this is a memoir and speaks from the heart. It is my story of these events. Anyone sufficiently invested in another narrative is free to provide their own and many people have already done just that.

Now it is my turn.

Chapter One

Planning the Birth of a Child: Hope and Reality

When we have babies without truly examining what we hold inside around birth, the least blip can lead to the entire plan unravelling. My mother's beliefs around birth were 'do what the doctor says' and when I had asked her if she knew what was happening during my birth, she snapped, "Of course! I knew to push when they told me to!" My birth ended with an episiotomy and forceps, from which I still bear a faint facial scar. My standard 1960s hospital crib photograph has my head carefully turned to hide the marks. Every year on my birthday, my mother became visibly uneasy and anxious, which I never understood until after she had died and I had babies. When I was eight, she achieved another pregnancy, but the baby was diagnosed with some kind of chromosomal disorder and the hospital performed a hysterotomy.[3] My mother was quietly distressed about her loss for the rest of her life. A year later, my sister was born via caesarean under a general anaesthetic which my mother described as significantly nicer. When your only vaginal birth experience is your legs in forceps, no support, people shouting to push, then cutting your vagina open with scissors and reaching inside you with huge metal tongs, this is unsurprising. Overall, her message was to do what the doctor says.

The legal arguments at the inquest dated the beginning of my 'fall' back to my decision to plan a homebirth with my first child. Though, in line with other ways in which I was constructed, they did not begin with the records from my midwife, who lived about ten minutes walk from our house. They began with the records of my transfer to hospital. After 24 hours of standard first time mother labour, my midwife told me my baby was 'stuck' and I needed to go to hospital and advocate for a caesarean. I did what she said.

When I was 21 and briefly, accidentally, pregnant, I read Sheila Kitzinger.[4] That pregnancy ended, as have many for me, in miscarriage, but I retained a fascination for birth from then on. I read and read years later when trying to conceive my first child. Two and a half years and two miscarriages later, I was finally pregnant with a sticky one. The more I read, the less I wanted anything to do with obstetrics. Women had begun writing about what we then called 'birth trauma' and as Kitzinger said, the memories of birth are with us for the rest of our lives. I wanted my memories to be of a birth in which my baby and I were respected, most of all. I now know for sure that the memories of birth last a lifetime and mine are not of birthing experiences where I have been respected. So I planned the homebirth, stayed home and, being a good girl who'd hired an expert in case of emergency, I did as I was told.

I naively believed that in what I thought was an hour of need, the hospital staff would respect me. I was wrong. As anyone who's planned a homebirth knows, transfer is almost always fraught. Over the years I've heard from only a handful of women for whom transfer was without punitive acts or abuse of some kind from physical assault to reporting a midwife whose actions had been totally fine. Most midwives are reported, after all, not by their clients but by bystanders. Vexatious reporting leading to immediate cessation of practice means women left without a midwife and a midwife who may lose all her equipment, phone and computer. Doctors who are sometimes reported over and over by patients, undergo no such judgment or loss, and famously dangerous doctors can go on plying an outrageous game for decades without the public being made safe from them.[5]

All that aside, it ended poorly for me with PTSD (post-traumatic stress disorder) and eventually suicidal feelings, which led me to seek help when my first child was six months old. I also saw a GP at this time because, you know, the campaigns are always "Feeling suicidal? Seek help from your GP!" My partner, baby and I attended the local doctor where he told me I had PND (post natal depression), and I said I didn't. Then he told me to look at the positives, which were that I was alive and so was my baby. I said I thought not dying was an impoverished goal of maternity care and surely we could do better. Then he told me I should seek treatment from a maternity hospital (at least not the one which harmed us), and rang to make me an appointment. I asked what this might consist of and he said they'd take my baby in another room and test me for various things and somehow help me to get over this. I observed that people taking my baby to another room was part of what caused this deep distress and trauma and I didn't feel doing it again would prove therapeutic. He didn't listen; he just went on with the 'you have PND' script. He finished our appointment by saying, "Come back and see me in a few weeks."

When we got home, I rang the hospital and cancelled the appointment. I never went back to that GP and he never contacted me to see if I was still alive. Considering one of the leading causes of death for women in the first year after childbirth is suicide,[6] he could have done better. But then my midwife had also failed me at that time. When I summoned up the courage to call her, a fortnight after the initial breakdown, she said, "Was it really that bad Janet?" Her advice at the time was for me to go back to the hospital that had harmed us and seek their care. I had a panic attack. How could anyone consider it helpful to go back to the people who'd done this to me as if they would make it ok? There is almost no recognition in the system that they even do this to us, so how would a maternity hospital deal with a woman showing up and asking for mental health help when she knew their philosophy and staff had caused the trauma? I've actually never gone back there, though I go past the hospital from time to time when I'm in Melbourne. It never gives me a good feeling.

It was these experiences which led me to feel like an epidemic of obstetric violence – which we then called birth trauma – really was as omnipresent as it had seemed when I planned to avoid it by birthing at home. And it made me think what must it be like for the women who aren't white, middle-class, educated and fairly assertive. I saw the mainstream birth advocacy groups around me, frightened to promote the only real model of one-to-one midwifery that existed, for fear of being seen as crazies. I did ask members of these groups why they didn't promote birthing outside of hospitals to women when they expressed concern about the way the system processes and treats women. The answer was usually something like: "We work for all women and we don't want to be seen to be pushing our own barrow." At that time, those groups were largely run by women who'd mostly or mainly birthed at home. They actually had no clue what it was like to be swept up in a misogynistic conveyor belt and seemed to feel little empathy. It was the old tension between working *with* the system (and legitimising its position as the arbiters of women's freedom), and working *outside* the system to create something by women for women. I fell into the latter camp and thus was born Joyous Birth, the Australian homebirth network.

Naively, I thought the existing groups would see Joyous Birth and the birth trauma group I started simultaneously, Accessing Artemis, as useful additions to the scene. None of them were tackling the trauma aspect, which in the middle of my own trauma seemed pretty clearly to be everywhere. None of them were saying aloud, "There is already a one-to-one midwifery option and it's available in your own home where you're the boss." So it seemed like a gap in the market, as the capitalists would say. I was motivated by never wanting to hear another woman's story of obstetric violence which she finished by saying, "I wish I'd known I could have birthed at home."

These were the days of the yahoo email lists, so that's what we used. Women joined up immediately in both groups, seeking support from both inside and outside Australia. I also attended some mainstream birth advocacy group meetings including one on the topic of birthing after a caesarean but again, the overall message was one of pacification rather than self-actualisation. I listened to well-meaning women, with their own trauma, describe to us that it doesn't matter how you birth so long as you're respected. This may be true in some senses but variations of birth do mean you can plan, but then must also make new decisions as birth unfolds. These groups pushed the idea that women could 'choose' to birth in the system and somehow achieve the outcome they most wanted, a vaginal birth after previous surgery, if they only used the right approach and tools. These ranged from birth plans (and how to produce them so they weren't offensive to hospital staff), to staying home until your babe was about to be born. They also included saying no to everything in the venue that might impede your plan or even taking baked goods when you went to have your baby (I kid you not, this is a serious suggestion).

The basic problem with all these approaches is the failure to acknowledge that this is a systemic, institutional denial of women's rights and the polar opposite of what is required for birth. Eventually it ends up, just like the system, in putting all the blame for the outcome on women. But it also gives women an out for when they go back to the same people who sliced them and end up with the same result. "I gave it my best shot, I hired a doula, I had a birth plan. And this time the surgery was much nicer." To invoke the spirit of Audre Lorde, these tools of the master were employed again and again – without a lot of luck, merely cementing the master's house, rather than dismantling it.[7]

Rights of Women First

It turns out other maternity advocacy groups weren't thrilled once they realised that the thrust of Joyous Birth was not midwives' rights in and of themselves, but women's autonomy from which all the rights would flow. I didn't articulate it in this way at the time. I was, in fact, fervently pro-midwives and their right to practise. While I have not shifted from that position, I have a lot more caveats in place around it now and a far more nuanced understanding of what's required. What women really lack is *autonomy* in our lives, and thus in our birthing as well. I did start saying early on in JB (we all call it JB) that if women's lives are better, then our birthing is better. Birth is a distillation and indication of women's overall rights in any society. We have rights on paper, which may well form the easier part of social change. What we don't have is *respect* in reality, just lip service about it. When we engage in the kinds of harm minimisation and impact amelioration which traditionally serves as birth advocacy, we cement the existing status quo. We can hold the best intentions possible, but without women's autonomy and personhood front and centre, none of it matters.

We started out admirably in Australia with birth advocacy being 'women and midwives together.' This is a noble and excellent aim. Midwives in the later twentieth century, who worked outside the system particularly, did see themselves as with the women. Midwife literally means 'with woman' and midwives as a group identified with women as a group, and saw the attainment of professional rights as desirable *in so far as they served the needs of women.*

Then the start of the twenty-first century saw the most open attacks on the whole enterprise of midwifery with the removal of insurance from privately practising midwives and the beginning of the wedge between women as a group and midwives as a group.[8] This wedge politics has been extraordinarily successful and women have been mostly co-opted under the original 'women and midwives together' banner to promote the professional rights of midwives even when they do not serve the rights of women. A triumph – and an international one – for obstetric ideology.

The opposition to midwifery has been carried out by doctors and their lobby groups, but also by the well-funded pharmaceutical companies and associated groups, for more than 200 years. While I am uncomfortable linking our present day circumstances to witch crazes, we can safely note that this is an ongoing attack with hundreds of years behind it.[9] The attempt to control midwives is at heart an attempt to control women. Professor Marjorie Tew detailed in *Safer Childbirth?* (1990) how doctors in the UK worked to make midwifery appear dangerous and we can see the same tactics here. What's bemusing to me is how despite it being so well-documented, we still fall for it. Doctors point to midwives having a lack of safety; governments and regulatory bodies begin to curtail women's rights to access the careproviders of their choosing; and the cycle continues. We followed, and continue to follow, this pattern in Australia. The push by career midwives (as opposed to vocational midwives) to professionalise by gaining the kind of kudos obstetricians attract, has harmed Australian women and our birthing. Governments use midwives to regulate women and when collective action by midwives could align them with women, and support women's autonomy, midwifery groups took what they perceived as a step forward for them, not us. And it is now 'them and us', sadly. Divide and rule has fixed the parameters for birthing women in uncomfortable and untenable places.

You would think that a tiny largely online group (though JB members did meet weekly in many places for some years as well) which represented fewer than 1% of the births in Australia would not pose a threat to the industrial obstetric complex. As a banner said at the time, "99% of births weren't enough for you?" But in the heady days of the early 2000s, Senate inquiries were a dime a dozen and homebirthing groups and women participated fiercely and directly in support of the rights of all women, wherever they birth, but particularly in the face of what was so obviously an attack on women choosing homebirth.[10] We wrote many submissions, letters, visited members of parliament including one Scott Morrison[11] who said women should not be allowed to birth at home. His opposition to abortion goes hand in hand with his belief that someone other than the birthing woman should be making the decisions about how and where we birth.

Individual midwives were picked off during this time including Lisa Barrett, a brilliant midwife who came to us from Britain and really galvanised women to fight from a science-based, rights-based corner. Despite being found in 2019 *not* guilty of manslaughter with regard to a stillbirth outside a hospital,[12] the loss of women like Lisa has been profound. The reality of birth, wherever you birth, is that some births end in loss. The rates of stillbirth in Australia have not changed much in decades and we have quite a high rate of stillbirth compared with some other western countries. Our homebirth stillbirth rates, however, have always been lower than those of the hospitals, a fact that no woman is ever given when she goes to her antenatal appointments in hospitals. The fact is that birth is as safe as life gets, as Harriette Hartigan once wisely observed,[13] and birth allowed to unfold to its own timetable is far less eventful than birth interfered with can ever be. We all know that tipping the birth's direction with inductions, drugs and time limits increases rates of further intervention and particularly those of surgeries, whether vaginal or abdominal. Obstetric propaganda being everywhere nowadays, we have all had our consent manufactured throughout our lives, so going to hospital is now the norm regardless of how poor the outcomes are in comparison with homebirth. It is not the magic of the venue, it is the normality of birth, and there is no 'normal' birth in hospitals. How could there be? We often say in the birth world that the same conditions required to get the baby in there, will get the baby out. We all make those "could you defecate in front of total strangers?" comparisons. But birth has become a victim of industrialisation as much as the next normal life event, from education to family life. Without some discourse to challenge it, women unsurprisingly follow the well-trodden path everyone around them follows. Unless we happen to come across other women modelling different ways to birth, which involve centring a birthing woman and her babe, why wouldn't we? You cannot be what you cannot see.

But why is all this relevant to me? Well, it's amazing how much disapproval and hatred one woman can attract when she stands for women in the face of an international movement to control women and profit from our bodies. I was a literal nobody who did a few TV and radio interviews, wrote occasional articles for journals, ran a homebirth group and refused to condemn women who birthed without midwives or doctors, in their own homes. Another birth advocate, who herself chooses to birth at home with her family, said to me once that she doesn't speak about that because it would lead the media to focus on that to the detriment of her work. Perhaps she was right. Certainly it's true that despite thousands of words on the benefit of midwifery care for those who choose it, advocating first and foremost for women's autonomy and our right to what's become freebirth, made it easy to paint me in that light. 'Price of belief may be a baby's life'[14] was a popular kind of headline in the months and years after my stillbirth because why bother to research the woman who needs slapping down in the moment? Despite writing pamphlets, papers, submissions, countless blog entries and attending meetings in support of women's right to midwifery, all that mattered was I also said women can birth at home without a midwife present if they so choose, and why shouldn't they? It is, after all, only if we envisage birth as something granted to us by others, that we can consider advocating for its naked form an affront.

Chapter Two

Birthing at Home

Back in the early 2000s, when midwife-assisted homebirth suddenly became more topical in the mainstream press, so too freebirth, or family birth, became more widely known.

Our culture of control over women means that the shock value of women birthing autonomously is on a par with those women who chained themselves to parliament houses for the privilege of voting. The politicised nature of birth, and the heavily contested zone of women's bodies, means that any choice outside of an external careprovider model is scrutinised, criticised and demonised. Those of us who birth in hospitals are seldom asked to justify our decision.

There are a number of broad reasons often given for those who choose freebirth – note that this is not the same as women speaking for themselves. Some reasons include the cost of private midwifery care, availability of midwifery care, fear of careproviders, or previous trauma. All of these are still coming to us via a paradigm which assumes the only model for birth to be one in which women seek external care provision. This argument posits that only 'damaged goods' or those without access to midwives would need or want to birth without an obstetric attendant, thus cementing the primacy of the external careprovider in birth. Our births are not defined in relation to us but by the cast attending us. For some women, some of these factors do come into play. For many women these are not factors which they consider when planning a birth. Those living in major cities, for instance, have little trouble locating independent midwives.

The pressures on independent midwives are well known to those of us who work in birth[15] and it cannot fail to be acknowledged as reprehensible that obstetricians who work without evidence or woman-centred care are favoured on every level over those who would seek to offer women something of benefit to them, their families and also the wider community. What some midwives fail to recognise, however, is that the very pressures on them from those bureaucracies which seek to stamp out homebirth, are filtering down to clients in a very real way via the regulating of mothers and midwives.[16] Some midwives clearly do recognise this and make deliberate decisions to pass on the impact of regulation to birthing women. The obstetric model of 'care with strings' is the one promoted by these bureaucracies. Women are forced to accept birthing under conditions that may indeed favour a midwife's continued access to registration, but do not support women to achieve the births they desire. However the end result is arrived at, some women are thus unable to find midwives to truly care for them and decide that they will be an autonomous consumer within the healthcare system and care for themselves.

Freebirth is thus not an attack on midwifery but for some women it is an indication that midwifery as it stands is unable to fulfil the needs of many consumers, myself among them. Perhaps rather than viewing freebirthing women (and those who support them) as another enemy, it would serve some careproviders well to use this information to reflect upon how to manage these issues without clients being affected. The use of freebirthing women's stories to promote midwives' campaigns for professional recognition is a misguided approach and only furthers the existing paternalism around birth. Midwives should be freely available to all women. To exploit some women's decisions to birth without a midwife in order to further a very different agenda does not seem a deeply considered strategy. Increased availability of midwives, desirable as it is, will not alter every woman's freebirth plans given the range of reasons women might choose freebirth in the first place. Nor should it, since women's right to choose within birth must be inviolable.

However a woman arrives at the decision to pursue freebirth, it almost always boils down to a desire for autonomy. Autonomy is not available to women in the hospital system and it is not available to all women choosing independent midwifery. In fact, it is generally not available to (nor is it pursued by many) women in our lives outside of birthing. But some women want to truly make their own decisions around their bodies, births and babies. This can only be a radical concept in a world where women are seldom supported in their basic rights to bodily integrity.

Imagining women with an automatic right to full autonomy is disturbing to many of us, acculturated as we are to believe that women are communal property, subject to the invasive gaze of authorities both public and private. It seems a difficult concept for careproviders who come from a background of normal socialisation and inherently misogynist training to grasp, but it is as difficult a concept for many women to grasp and those who do are a (maligned) minority. Some women even recognise that it is their response to the client/careprovider dynamic which leads them to choose autonomous birth and thus circumvent their own socialisation to hand over their power. Careproviders might find their own personal and professional satisfaction concomitantly increased by taking similar steps.

There is no way for us to describe women who birth outside obstetric systems in the west without the lens of normalised surveillance coming to bear. I am using the term devised by Professor Marjorie Tew here. She called antenatal care, 'antenatal surveillance' in her book, *Safer Childbirth?: A Critical History of Maternity Care.*[17] She unequivocally demonstrated that the move from home to hospital birth in Britain decreased women's safety in birth considerably. She pointed to two clear places in her survey which showed that World War Two improved women's nutrition (because the main eater in the house was away) which was one pillar of an improvement in birthing outcomes. The second good outcome for women in Britain post the move to hospitals was when most of the doctors were away at the war. But our discourse around birth does not reflect these observations.

As Professor Tew wrote: "When the history is told, it becomes clear that at no time in the past or present and in no country have medical interventions made childbirth safer for most mothers and babies."[18]

She also notes, "By contrast, many interventions undoubtedly cause positive harm."[19] She quotes an anonymous colleague of William Silverman, considered by many to be the pioneer of what we call 'evidence-based medicine', saying:

> The most recent history of perinatal medicine abounds with instances in which belated controlled trials eventually revealed that the apparent benefits of some widely acclaimed treatment had merely disguised the real extent of its tragic consequences.[20]

In 2007, I began calling rebel birthers 'autonomous consumers'[21] because the term 'unassisted birth' still implies that birthing with paid attendants is the norm from which autonomous consumers differ and the label 'freebirth' as developed by women, doesn't really have a lot of meaning outside its own milieu. Other women use the term 'family birth', which I also like because it captures what women have done for eons.

So when a woman like me, white, middle-class and educated, chooses a birth with her family or friends in attendance over one with a registered state-approved careprovider, the only language available is that of pathology.

Although I was publicly pregnant on the internet and in my daily life, during the inquest I was accused of having concealed my pregnancy. Because I chose to avoid institutional pregnancy surveillance, I was put under the 'concealed pregnancy' umbrella;

the taint of a woman keeping herself private from society and institutions. The year my baby was born, the New South Wales Ombudsman's report into *Reviewable Child Deaths* described my baby and an anonymous 14-year-old foster child's baby thus:

> Two infants were born following either concealed pregnancy or unrecognised pregnancy and unassisted birth, and did not appear to have been provided with the care and attention necessary to sustain life. Both babies died less than a day after birth. The cause of death for the two infants is undetermined.[22]

But only one of those births merited an inquest. The pregnancy and birth of a demonstrably competent 40-year-old woman merited the public investigation of an inquest while the obvious systemic failure of a 14-year-old child in state care made pregnant while in foster care, did not.

My baby was born dead and I do not know about the young girl's baby, so again, the comment "dying less than a day after birth" means very little but implies inaction or neglect on my part, and hers, as if we watched our babies die in front of us. Following this up with "the cause of death … is undetermined" would then seem to contradict the first statement of death being due to our neglect. These are the ways in which a weight of implications and blame for the loss of a baby is brought down on mothers – and yet to most people these are neutral descriptors. For me, blaming women for sad outcomes is the baseline for the discourse around stillbirth.

A 'concealed pregnancy' is considered on a par with pregnancy denial where a girl or woman ignores or denies the fact of her pregnancy. It's written about as a mental disorder. It is often conflated with what is called 'cryptic pregnancy', which generally means a woman unaware she is pregnant until birth occurs but is sometimes confused with 'false pregnancy', being a woman who believes herself to be pregnant despite evidence to the contrary.

Estimates for the conflated pregnancy concealment and denial can vary from 1 in 400 to 1 in 2500 depending on the source. Studies on these start from a baseline assumption of unsurveilled pregnancy as innately dangerous to mother and baby. They stem from our normalised expectation that obstetrically managed pregnancy and birth is superior. I would argue, however, that this is a mix of cognitive dissonance, with our consent manufactured on a grand scale, as well as primal invisible fears that uncontrolled women are a danger to society. One meta-analysis of 669,876 women's births, showed no improvement in outcomes for women or babies who attended hospital antenatal surveillance.[23] In fact, a Finnish study[24] of 57,000 women showed the more antenatal surveillance, the poorer the outcome in terms of low birth weight, premature infants, more caesarean sections, instrumental delivery and also the highest rates of induction of labour. Obviously these are not the only tools women use when deciding on a place of birth but it can serve us well to look outside the usually considered if we are to find our own paths.

Chapter Three

Birthing My Daughter

The Journey

Teetering on the edge
not like those elephants on string
more like a drop of ocean
suspended over an abyss—
Waiting to roll down the inside
to the volcano
Slowly at first
but gathering pace
until engulfed in the lava
seeking an exit

But then
when least expected
the lull

Then the universe beckons
Arms, breasts, belly
all floating
whirling through space

held by the moon's pull
and the sun's rush
Epona's horses
churn a path
through the world
and set free the babe at last

Maybe not
like this at all
for each babe calls for its birth
You will gather yourself
and be the guide
The rock
the slippery path
beloved   almighty   required

~

May 2009

Imagine you are 39, unexpectedly pregnant with your third child who was a surprise after a fertility history normally involving long, tiring attempts to conceive over a number of years. Imagine the delight of your older children for whom this baby is both an unknown and a gift providing hours of conversation and growth and is coincidentally the exact distance from number two child, that number two child was from number one. Imagine some spotting, the first pregnancy you ever had spotting in but then getting past that, into the months of nausea and exhaustion and then into the bliss of the middle of pregnancy with a curvaceous bump and the lessening of that nausea. The belly grows and grows, friends offer support, a blessingway and then into hibernation and withdrawal from most of the world. Working up till a week before the babe is born, you drag yourself around with a wonky clunking pelvis, two energetic older children and the bittersweet knowledge that this is the last pregnancy and thus to be treasured, but also a sense of relief since pregnancy and birth have always been complex affairs in your life.

The first birth ended in surgery which was not lifesaving and nearly became life ending as it was processed amidst a lack of support and the world's opposition to the notion that careproviders do not always provide care but can also bring pain, suffering and violence to bear on a birth. The second birth was long and physically gruelling, directly after a betrayal and withdrawal of expected midwife care, which then required a transfer to hospital to obtain medical care that my careprovider should have provided. Then months (and years) of gossip and speculation and character assassination as your life and motives were picked over. This birth, you decide, will be different so you make plans, organise, buy the supplies time prevented being purchased last time. Spend time thinking things through, knowing that this is the right decision for you and your family. After weeks of labourish activity in your body, go into labour.

This is hard labour. It hurts. There is little labour trance, there is processing, talking, a little crying. There are children who must be cared for and who find some parts of their altered mother distressing. The usual times of humour, extreme bodily functions and the even more extreme good will of the friend who cleans them up. Day passes, night falls and you know the baby will be born that night, cutting in half the time of this labour in comparison with the last, but still a good hefty 24 hours will have passed in this state. Pushing pushing pushing, why does the baby not help? Pushing pushing pushing, will my lungs be born with this baby? Snap into awareness, demand a light goes on overhead. A head appears, phew. Dreading restitution, waiting. No restitution, decide to help the baby, push, push, ease ease, ow ow ow. Baby born, scooped up by daddy.

Slow motion ensues. Baby still. Baby limp. Baby perfect. No cry, no movement, no breath, no eye contact. No protest at leaving womb comfort and swimming into cool air. Calm ensues. You call your baby in, nothing. Triple O is called, CPR starts on a chair while you still kneel in the pool and unreality takes over. Men arrive in blue puffy pants with masses of equipment. The placenta falls out of you, the cord is cut, the bond is severed. The men in blue pump, blow and talk esoteric language to one another. One two three, hefted out of the pool, can't walk, bleeding, end up on the couch naked. Veins jabbed, questions asked, blood pressure taken, cannula inserted. "Can I go in the ambulance with her?"

"No." She is taken.

More questions, more bleeding. Turn around. Police? Police up the hall, in the loungeroom? What? No time to worry, hefted onto bed and wheeled out. Three ambulances? Four police cars? Forensic bus? No time to think, stay focused, breathe through afterpains and sore body. Morphine, more measuring of blood pressure. Conversations over your head. "Should I say she has three children or two on the paperwork?" Are you really that fucking tactless?

Reassure anxious partner whose heart can be heard beating over the noise of the engine, "She'll probably be intubated so prepare yourself for her to be sedated and not looking too good." Don't say, "She's dead, she's not coming back" because that will make it true and you're not ready to admit to it yet aloud. Hug the knowledge close to your chest because it is all you have. And some hope.

Arrive at the hospital. Police? That's weird. Wheeled past, into tiny cubicle, people asking questions, nice ambulance officer still helping out. Finally shoved in wheelchair, wheeled into emergency where tiny baby is surrounded by layers of strangers of which we are just another pair to this situation. Declared dead. Reassured that it looks like SIDS. Explain she's just been born and that makes it a stillbirth. (Idiot.) Holding still baby. Can't cry. Can't look in her face in case it shows distress, or accuses me of betrayal. People coming, going, wheeled into cubicle. Can't be alone with her? Can't have a room? What's going on? More police.

Time stops. Oh baby. Look at the curve of your limbs, the round belly, your soft head with all that hair, more hair than other babies I've made. Oh you look like your sister. So much, nearly too much. I will see the cast of your face on her for weeks to come. Put your skin to mine, still warm, so soft. Nearly too soft to touch. People again. Buzzing around. More questions, offer appropriate answers, use technical jargon, something familiar at last, talk about birth.

Police again, talking to partner, hanging around, talk starts of the baby being taken from you. Incomprehensible right now and now there is only now, there is not five minutes ago, not five minutes hence, just now. Push thought of baby taken to the back of the mind. Camera, photos, tubes covering baby's face, bruises from resuscitation, tubes and sticky things on her perfect little body, staff won't remove them because they're evidence. Evidence of what? What is happening? I hold her and kiss her; her father holds her and kisses her. Aunt, cousin, other aunt, holding, crying, kissing. Clothes appear. Putrid pink shite, she is dressed. Better clothes appear, she is redressed. More photos. Nurse warning again that she has to be taken from me. Finally I cry. No no no. Don't take her. She's all I have to show for this pregnancy, this birth, this life right now. She is not yours to take, she is not going in a police car, in a fridge who knows where. Don't take her. No no no.

Hand her over. Cry cry. Howl. Oh goddess the pain, not another child taken from me. My first was taken out of spite to show the homebirther who's boss. My second I kept safe. My third taken by the state. You can't fight The Man. Numb knowing she's gone. Cry and cry. Wrong wrong wrong. Hold ugly stripey blanket that smells of her. Bury face in it. Listen to staff treating patients in other cubicles, listen to man next door diagnosed with pneumonia. Cry more. House being searched? What? Children removed to friend's house? What? "Agree to search, we'll get a warrant anyway." Partner and sister go to be with older children, hers and ours. Oh god how do we tell them? Unreality. Empty arms. Lie down, hold blanket and inhale, she's still here somewhere.

Wheeled to a room. Can't go home, house locked up, police inside it. Can't walk. Need to catch my breath, maybe a private room where I can just be for a moment. Tell sisterfriend not to leave. I don't want to wake up with no uterus. She knows. Midwife on duty asks where the baby is? "She's dead," I say and bury my face in the blanket. It still smells of her. Inhale. She's here again. No, she's gone with the police. And her placenta? Gone. What's happening?

Shower. Wee. Brain keeps moving body regardless of the filleted fish of my soul. Midwife keeps saying birth is a sports injury, apply ice. Um no thanks. Lie down, aching, so much pain. Phone rings. (Phone rings?) "Hello this is the Coroner's office, your child will have a postmortem performed this afternoon. Ok?"

Gather thoughts. "What? No. Her father doesn't even know, I can't just tell him, we need to be together to process this information."

"You have to agree to the postmortem."

Head reeling. "Well, what else can I do?"

"You can challenge it. In the Supreme Court. After it's done. Do you have any questions?"

"How can I ask you questions when I have no information and no idea what or why this is happening?"

More inane conversation. PM on hold at least till I can talk to partner.

Lie down. Try to rest. Effort of will, shut out crying babies in every other room on this floor.

People walk in. Detectives. More questions. Why am I being difficult about the postmortem? Why am I obstructing them? What?

Explain again. Slowly. Wild-eyed lying in bed with officers standing near me. Nursing Unit Manager between them and me. If only she were much much larger. Keep explaining, it's not to be difficult, it's not to hide anything, it's that my baby was just born and now she's gone and her father is not in our home because you're searching it and I don't know how my other children are and now you're telling me I'm being difficult? Eventually they seem to get it but are unimpressed with my tenacity. The PM is put off till a few days away. Luckily a weekend interceded for me because no one else was going to. The power of Saturday, thank you. Told I can see my baby at the morgue the next day. I'm allowed to see her. Allowed. My baby.

They leave. They take sisterfriend. I'm alone. Phone rings. People in and out. Nice surgeon. Another woman, "Would you like to be part of a study on stillbirth?" Fuck off. Keep being polite, keep being nice, everyone's just doing their job and most of them are being considerate. Sister arrives and minds the space. I sleep. I sleep through the roaring babies, the phone is switched off. Blood pressure is left alone. More people wander in and out. Father visits. He's beside himself with discomfort. Makes himself busy Doing. Offers food, drink, goes on errands. Awake again. Hours later, time passes, is it afternoon? Long day so far. Wheeled down to car. Tears run silently down my face. I'm in the grief bubble where other people look so normal and my life has cracked open. Father stands next to the car, not looking at me, not speaking to me. He can't trust himself to not break down so he can't bear to look at me. I look at the fluffy slippers, close my eyes, wear my glasses since my sunglasses were at home. I had them on labouring in the backyard a lifetime ago. Drive home. Children, partner, sisterfriend, house tidied after search. Post on forums. Cry cry cry till I look like a prize fighter. Sleep. Thank goddess for exhaustion.

Chapter Four

> "It's of no use to look back and say, 'I should have been different'. At any given moment, we are the way we are, and we see what we're able to see. For that reason, guilt is always inappropriate."
>
> Charlotte Joko Beck, *Nothing Special* (1993)

The Aftermath

I think the word most commonly associated with stillbirth, unlike other deaths, is guilt. In my opinion, guilt is the main acceptable expression of grief around stillbirth. Hospital pamphlets and well-meaning counsellors often assure women that there's nothing they could have done, that stillbirth is random and that guilt is unnecessary. We are so uncomfortable with death in Australian mainstream society and I should so dearly love to see all of us able to embrace death as part of life, however agonising the loss we face.

It is perhaps a bit of a contradiction to suggest guilt as a response in the first place while simultaneously assuring us we don't need to feel it. If we don't need to feel it, why suggest it? My observation is that guilt remains a kind of trope, shorthand or cipher through which the wider world can manage the agony of stillbirth without addressing the true nature of its complexity. The idea is that women can use it as a recognised symbol of this kind of loss. Many of our responses are cast under the guilt umbrella when we may actually feel much more complicated emotions and pain. For me, the visceral trauma of my loss was akin to being emotionally flayed alive and the raw flesh pressed against the screaming universe. I said, at the time, I wanted to piss, shit, vomit and bleed all over the earth to somehow externalise the indescribable experience of being both life giver and human shroud to a loved child.

When that loss occurs at home, which pundits and doctors always suggest (despite evidence to the contrary) is the place most likely for stillbirth to occur, women then have a different experience. Some of us are still told that there's nothing we could have done, but the overall message is that the key thing you should have done was to have your baby in a hospital. In reality, loss occurs in all models of care and we still don't know why most losses occur. I have observed a keen sense of guilt in women regardless of where they birthed. What I have also observed is a series of contradictions around this. Women birthing in hospitals aren't immune to this narrative of maternal 'fault' wherever it appears, so the signposting of fault in one group of mothers doesn't necessarily translate to the relieving of guilt in others.

We are told that hospitals are the only safe place to birth and that there is a substantial body count associated with birthing outside of institutions. In reality, given that more than 99% of births happen in hospitals here, so do 99% of the stillbirths. We have ways of shutting down the discourse around that though, and the names or addresses of women who experience losses in hospitals seldom come to light. The nursing staff, midwives and doctors are only named under exceptional circumstances. They are afforded appropriate confidentiality. Those of us who experience loss at home don't always have these niceties applied to us.

The Law Intervenes on Postmortem

The day my baby was mostly cremated was a week after her birth. I say 'mostly' as she had a skull full of wadding because her brain had been removed and kept by the pathologists. Her spinal cord was also missing. A few days later, at the end of the day after the fires were switched off, her brain and spinal cord were cremated to be put in with the rest of her ashes. I was told after the fact that they kept some samples, though I was not told of what those comprised. I had little idea what exactly the postmortem might entail and it was nauseating to discover even her tiny vagina had been cut into. I assume that in the move from the morgue at Glebe to the new premises at Lidcombe, if not before, those remaining traces of my baby would have been destroyed. A stillbirth at home can mean that your baby is considered 'evidence' and you have no right to decide whether or not a postmortem occurs. Parents in hospitals can find themselves pressured to have, or not have, a postmortem. But at home, if the police and coronial staff deem it necessary, no permission is required. When I asked if the postmortem could wait until her father knew it was happening, the senior investigating officer told me it couldn't and that I could challenge it in the Supreme Court later if I wished. He also intimated that my questioning was being interpreted as oppositional and could be considered an attempt to pervert the course of justice.

Another woman, reporting to me about the issue of a postmortem for her own baby, said that the hospital staff told her they could do one if she wanted one, but that in many cases of stillbirth, an 'answer' is never found. She said:

> I decided that because she appeared 'normal' morphologically, and there was no obvious reason for her demise (like a cord knot) that it is likely the postmortem wouldn't show up anything. I didn't want her body to be autopsied. They took my bloods instead, to see if they could see any reason for her death.[25]

One more woman, whose baby was born at home after which they transferred him to hospital, said:

> The Paediatric Registrar spoke with us about our options for testing and an autopsy. We declined. I asked for the placenta to be returned to me (with hopes to bury it under a tree like his older brother's) and I was advised that due to the testing that was going to be completed on it, that I wouldn't be getting it back. Which sucked.[26]

There is a new idea being floated whereby the federal government pays for postmortems on stillborns.[27] I have never been under the impression that it is the lack of funding that leads to families deciding not to pursue postmortems. It is generally accepted that in around 50% of stillbirths there is no discernible reason for the loss even with a postmortem so what this drive seeks to achieve is unclear to me. Will it result in greater pressure on hospital birthing women to accept a postmortem for their babies? I don't know. Australian hospitals have a higher rate of stillbirth than hospitals in comparable western countries and this is considered a bit of a mystery by most people. Maybe the Select Committee on Stillbirth Research and Education[28] will speak to that in a genuine way but I don't know if that's possible given our inability to look honestly at our maternity care system.

None of these facts, easily accessible and from government sources, form part of any media discourse around the place of birth. Susie O'Brien in the tabloid Melbourne newspaper *The Herald-Sun* wrote in 2012, "Around 700 women across Australia give birth at home and in my opinion that's 700 too many."[29] And Mia Freedman said about freebirth, "the idea does my head in."[30]

What Happens When a Baby is Stillborn?

My baby was born at home in my study, in the same spot her sister had been born two years and eight months previously. When she was born and didn't immediately breathe, we went into emergency mode and began 'calling her in', as we say in homebirths. Sometimes a slow-to-get-going baby will come to itself when the mother speaks to them, brushes their face and strokes their chest. When that didn't work, we moved onto CPR, which was performed by me and also a friend. Video of the

CPR was viewed in court and experts agreed it was performed correctly. My partner called an ambulance. Five police cars, three ambulances and a forensic truck arrived before we'd even left for the hospital and prior to my baby being declared dead.

In the hospital, while the staff were very kind to me, the police were always present. I was not allowed to be alone with my baby, nor was I given access to the stillbirth rooms at Royal Prince Alfred in Sydney (RPA) which were located at the entrance to the antenatal corridor at that time. I was in an emergency cubicle largely undressed, visible to police through gaps in the curtains. This was just prior to the advent of groups like Heartfelt, which takes bereavement photographs in hospitals[31] but they usually have a camera on the ward for such occasions so some photos were taken of me that are truly horrible. I was forbidden to remove the resuscitation tubes and other medical paraphernalia from my daughter because it was also evidence and she was just beginning to cool and stiffen. One staff member advised me it would be good if I handed her over to the police soon because the next shift was coming on and included a member who wouldn't be nice to me.

Handing her over was one of the hardest things I'd ever had to consider in my life and I simply couldn't physically do it. So I handed her to her father who handed her to a staff member who handed her to a police officer. She was taken in their storage equipment to the morgue at Glebe where an officer who became the Senior Investigating Officer (SIO) 'identified' her for their paperwork. She was put in a locker there. It still causes me pain that a stranger could be said to have identified my baby.

I was wheeled to the postnatal ward where I was greeted by a midwife who asked where the baby was, since nowadays it is no longer normal to remove the baby from a newly birthed mother. The next few hours are a bit foggy for me. I know some things that happened and can be verified from records. I know some things that happened and cannot be verified because they happened for me and are thus not dignified by note taking. I know some things that didn't happen at all – but for which I was condemned later in court.

Betrayal

A woman who knows said to me the other day that the work of women's liberation is to survive the betrayal of other women. Even for my nihilistic tastes, this was bleak. And yet as I contemplate it, this sad point does speak to me. I find it is the betrayals around my birth and the inquest that sting and still cause me pain. Without a critique of women's self-hatred, I think I would implode, or explode. The compounded trauma of these years is never far from me.

Even today as I've tried to write this I've heard a friend has had a stillbirth. I've also had a message and an email from the friend who is checking if I can afford the transcript of the inquest. I promptly fell in a heap. When I could stop keening and stand up, I went to the deck. I swayed like a labouring woman and did more silent keening because my children are home. I lay on the deck in the sun with the wind whipping the birches. "I am the tree," I said experimentally, though which tree it is that moors in toffee and waves branches through sludge, I do not know. I am that tree though. And I prayed valiantly not to throw up. Gorge rising again to type that. This is trauma and no doubt familiar to all who experience it.

After my baby was born and taken by police to the morgue at Glebe, I was allowed to see her the following day. I had cried throughout the whole night. In the morning my daughter cried because my face was so swollen I was unrecognisable. We went to the morgue, her father and I. Walking in, a total stranger shows us to a room which I think in retrospect may have been intended for counselling. They probably wheel adult corpses in, but my baby can be carried, in arms, from the fridge. I can't stand up any longer. Legs buckling I sit on the floor. Her father sobs beside me. I have spent all night crying over and over I'm sorry I'm sorry I'm sorry though he doesn't blame me because he is decent and knows life can be shit.

We undress her because babies should be naked with mothers. They have removed the tubes now that they have taken them as evidence. Later I learn there are photos of her but I didn't know then. I talk to her; people take photos. We have so many photos later.

As I start to calm down and the new scenario normalises for me, I chat to the forensic psychologist. If I'd read a pamphlet,

I'd have known that families of grieving people have one assigned to them. I didn't read the pamphlet for about three years though, so I don't know quite what I thought she was other than a counselling type person? I asked for my placenta so we could make placenta prints.[32]

No one had ever asked that in the history of the Department of Forensic Medicine so there was no process for it but eventually someone said yes and the psychologist brought it in a bucket for me. I keep building rapport and she says she's had two sons but never seen her placenta.

My heart goes out to women at all times but in that cracked open time I'd have given any woman the clothes off my whipped back and she was no different. So I gave her a tour of the cord, two normal looking arteries and a vein, the different parts, a quick story about consuming some raw at my previous birth. And we did the prints. She commented to me that I was kind, loving and generous and I said, "Thank you, that's who I try to be." At the end of our second meeting, when I was again allowed to hold my baby before she was cut, I felt enough rapport to hand my baby straight to her rather than going through the intermediary, her father, as I had at our first meeting.

But then, when we were preparing for the inquest, a mysterious comment surfaced which I had apparently made. My barrister asked what terrible thing I'd said. I had no idea. But according to the forensic psychologist, I had made a terrible comment at one point, which was so very terrible she couldn't write it down. She could, however, telephone the police and tell them the comment.

The police verbally relayed the comment to the Coroner who also was so very shocked he couldn't record the comment. The forensic psychologist finished her part in the police brief by saying it was important I didn't find out she'd passed on my comment to the police because she felt I had lost faith in authorities and would convince my 'followers' to refuse to cooperate with 'medico-legal authorities'. To this day I'm not sure I understand what a medico-legal authority is but I can promise I have no such sway over anyone let alone any 'followers'. I can't even get my dogs to come to me in the park so the idea I have anyone doing my bidding is ludicrous.

But it strikes me as a terribly unethical act and I was shocked to the core when I discovered it three years later. If I'd read the pamphlet, would I have been more shocked? Would I have expected some kind of confidentiality from someone caring for us? I don't know. And the mystery of what I said remains. My best guess is that when speaking to my sister, who had come to the morgue to see my baby, I made some crack in poor taste as we probably all do under terrible strain and in a morgue, as my sister and I share a familial sense of dark humour when death is involved. Would not a forensic psychologist have seen and heard everything under the sun grieving families might do? Would she not feel a sense of compassion or empathy? Was my pre-existing status as a 'dangerous woman' overriding all she had seen from me when I cared for her in the midst of my own loss? It is interesting how much a Bad Mother can never throw off those shackles of supposed ill-intent even when the evidence is before someone and she herself had remarked upon my character so positively. It was not the first, nor the last betrayal.

Pathologising Women

I strongly feel that a stillbirth at a freebirth pulls together two important pillars for the analysis of pregnant women: the pathologising of 'concealed pregnancy' and the belief that pregnancy and birth without surveillance are inherently unsafe. But also that women have no right to choose their place of birth, or attendants, unless within those boundaries approved by obstetrics. Both of these define the women involved as a danger to our babies, probably mentally ill, and potentially also a danger to society. Unsurveilled women, pregnant or not, are a threat to the good order of a patriarchy. While legally we do not have personhood of the foetus in Australia, it is clear that we have a culture of it in the medical system and also in the minds of many people. I have often remarked that Australians are largely in favour of women's access to abortion but that they cannot tolerate the notion that women might freely choose how or where to birth. Pregnancy indicates that sex has occurred which makes us fair game in the minds of most people and leads to intrusive behaviours such as touching pregnant women.

I was pathologised from go to whoa. A few of the examples include the ambulance officer whose witness statement to police described me as having a personality disorder. His evidence for this was that as he entered my birthing room, I was holding my baby in a position he considered strange and which in breast-feeding circles we call a football hold. I then handed him my baby, which he interpreted as a lack of attachment and affect on my part. His testimony also led to Counsel Assisting criticising me for risking the lives of ambulance officers by having my birth pool in a small room which apparently could have led to them falling in. This was my study, which also contains a number of bookshelves, the spare futon bed, my desk and several chairs. It's not a tiny room. From my point of view, we discontinued CPR when the ambulance officers walked into the room. Since the people I perceive as experts in CPR were then present, I handed them my child. What is the converse to this situation? How would he have interpreted my actions had I held onto her and refused to hand her over? Would that have been me denying my baby emergency care? Which personality disorder is covered by that? My barrister successfully argued for this evidence to be disregarded and not to be presented in court.

~

I was not made for this time

Death by bureaucracy
should not be my fate

I was made for horses
freedom
a battle on equal terms

Warrior women are now
Aberrant
Abnormal

Crones dismissed
Where we should rule
And advise

So what to do with this spirit
this soul of power
in a time of evil banality?

I wish I knew

Police repeatedly described me as obstructive. When my barrister asked for examples of this, none could be found. Despite speaking to police in the hospital at their request, participating in a police interview three weeks later and not putting any barriers between them and the many hours of searching our home, I was still considered uncooperative. To whit, the means by which I was subpoenaed. Given that the police knew I had a solicitor acting for me and thus I would be attending the inquest, the SIO made a point of issuing me with a subpoena. First he attended my home during a weekday. He called my by then ex-partner at work to ask my whereabouts. I was in the city with our homeschooled children. He did not leave me a card saying he'd called and could I contact him. Then he attended my home on a Saturday evening. Again I failed to be present and again, he telephoned my ex-partner and asked him why I was 'avoiding police'. My ex told him I wasn't and called me to let me know. I then contacted my solicitor to ask if this was reasonable and he confirmed it wasn't. On the Monday morning, I rang the station and left a voicemail for the SIO saying, "I will be home until 1 p.m. today if you wish to serve me." He turned up, I opened the door and took receipt of the subpoena. As usual, he gave me a withering look of disapproval.

The SIO had kicked that off three years previously in the hospital and then at my police interview. Like a criminal, I was taken in by the custody officer and cautioned. Then I was taken, with my then solicitor, down in a lift and into a windowless interrogation room. I believe my phobia of flying, which developed after this time, dated from this experience. My fight or flight reflexes have never been so present and I have never fought so hard against them until the inquest itself.

I remember every detail of clinging onto the shabby office chair in the custody sergeant's office, staring at my shoes and willing my legs to keep me seated when I wanted to run away from the danger very fast indeed. I was asked questions in the recorded interview which clearly showed to me the problem of having police ask questions about a normal, physiological process and with no understanding at all of birth. The questions sounded to me like he'd quizzed the wife over breakfast that morning and maybe drawn on a few pamphlets from when they were having kids. They included hard hitters like, "So most women in

Australia when they're pregnant, they hire an obstetrician and give birth in hospital but you don't."

Silently I pondered a response to this non-question by tossing around the fact that most women, in fact, simply go to hospital and that the hiring of a private obstetrician is a minority pursuit. I ended up answering, "No."

He also asked me some revealing questions like, "What does Trevor do?" though he never asked what I did. And the memorable question, "Is Trevor the father of all the children?" This went along with, "Was this baby a planned pregnancy?" It was clear in his view, that I was to blame for her death.

Chapter Five

The day before

Inhabit the space
when I can barely inhabit myself
Heart thudding tugging
to be free of this body.
Last coffee drunk before tomorrow's coffee.
Breathe slow to make each breath
not the last one.
Before tomorrow
blue sky beautiful.
Dead baby still not here.
Still not three nor playing with her siblings.
They ask often what she would be doing.
She is always reckoned in the family sums.
always the jagged hole in the black ice
of my heart.
The tears on my face right now even in public

Grief doesn't tidy away like socks
or even hide in the third drawer down
in the kitchen where the other mystery items lie.

Discomfort clear on the faces around me.
Distancing to avoid the fumes of my sour grief
peer at me through laced fingers.
No bargaining keeps relentless death at bay.
Best to stop turn face embrace.
This will be my lifelong relationship.
Who is brave enough to witness our nuptials?[33]

The Inquest

A packed courtroom including media greeted me on my first day in court. Several narratives were running simultaneously by this point. The Coroner had refused to hold a jurisdiction hearing which is one of the few essential legal steps around holding an inquiry. It is required that evidence be produced and examined to decide whether or not the case fits the remit of the Coroner. It is required that a baby be born alive in what's called 'the Born Alive rule'. There is no evidence my baby was born alive which makes me thus not to be blamed for her death. However, inquests into homebirth stillbirths are political and women must be punished. This is why we say 'death by homebirth' because regardless of the cause of death, or even if it's unknown, the findings are always that birthing at home caused the death of the baby.

Counsel Assisting gave the opening address which detailed all my sins and which the media dutifully copied down and printed.[34] Naturally, the media did not appear the day I was cross-examined. My own words weren't needed for this process.

By the time we got to court, I had been taught how to be cross-examined which was just as well since a lot of questions were a bit weird, quite frankly. There was a peculiar fascination with my books and writing via my blog and forums. "You have a lot of books," was an early one. The police had photographed and videoed my bookshelves. Photos of my bookshelves were put on the wall of the courtroom and I was quizzed about their contents.

"And what are these books?"

"Australian domestic architecture."

"And these?"

"Irish history …?"

"And these?"

"Birth and parenting."

"And have you read them all?"

"No."

My online activity was examined too. During the inquest, a post I had scheduled some time before popped up and there was much teeth sucking and displeasure from the Coroner at its content.

The problem faced by Counsel Assisting was making me out to be sufficiently knowledgeable so that they could say I was wantonly neglectful, yet ignorant enough to say I was horrifyingly uninformed and therefore also neglectful.

Looking for the Witch Mark

I alluded earlier to how I don't like to use the term 'witch hunt' when describing what is done to us around homebirth in Australia. I would suggest, however, that use of similar tactics to force me to appear naked in a video shown repeatedly during the inquest, do bring to mind looking for the witch mark. Like a lot of homebirthing women, I had a video of my birth. During the police search, the video and stills camera were both taken and copied in full to be entered into evidence. Stills from before I'd even become pregnant formed part of the brief as did my very naughty staged joke book-burning of some horrible anti-baby parenting books. These were described as "book burning by unknown female" who is my sister. We were having a bonfire in the backyard for solstice. These images went towards building my character as a danger to society. But the video of my birth was used to punish me, I have no doubt.

In preparation to go to court, I had needed to watch this video of my daughter being born and my initial attempts to clear her airways, call her in, drain her and so on. I hadn't watched that video until I sat in my solicitor's office. I had to watch it a number of times while talking to him about what we could see. He had needed me to tell him what I was doing and I needed to see the video to do that because I had no memories of that time except some physical and emotional memories. So it was almost like watching someone else. That day was a profound and painful one for me. In order to prepare myself I had gone into the city early and walked down to the harbour, through the Botanic Gardens, stopped briefly in the Art Gallery, then headed on over to my solicitor's office. I felt a galvanising, powerful sense of acceptance as I walked because I needed to breathe and just embrace what was about to happen or the pain would overcome me. I also had a really powerful sense of forgiveness towards the Crown Solicitors and the Coroner because they knew I would have to see this video and I knew they would play it in court as part of my punishment.

They did. And I had to watch it and so did her father, my attending friend and all the journalists, court officers, supporters and any other random people who popped in that very full day. Imagine yourself naked, on a large screen, being shown to strangers against your will. Discomforting, isn't it?

The first witness on the first day was a friend who'd been assured that she wouldn't be forced to view the video of me birthing my baby and beginning CPR. They put the video on. I left the room because I didn't want what I said to be tainted by anything she said. Then they put the video on again and cross-examined my ex-partner on it. I was called and it was played again, for me to be cross-examined about my actions in the video. All this in an open court, with media and mobile phones. I don't know about you but one of the many reasons I birth at home is to retain the kind of privacy that supports normal birthing. Having police, witnesses (some who knew me and some who didn't), court officials, attendees (some of whom were supportive and most who weren't), lawyers and anyone else who felt like it, viewing my naked body over and over had a definite ring of voyeurism to it.

Normally, I don't watch the videos of me birthing. There is, for me, something bizarre about witnessing myself and hearing those scenes and I've never done it despite the previous children's labours and births being recorded. That's their property, in my mind, and I'll never watch the videos. So forcing me to watch me giving birth felt like a deep insult to me both psychically and emotionally, which I suspect was the intent whether conscious or not. As my barrister remarked, if this was a trial rather than an inquest, the video would have completely exonerated me of any wrongdoing since even the most hostile experts present agreed the CPR performed was perfectly correct.

~

My mother-in-law came to stay for that week and cared for the kids while I went to court every morning, collected in a cab by their father. The first night I came home late after dinner with other attendees and they were both asleep. My littler one was asleep on the floor. I lay on the floor to spoon her and sobbed. My mother-in-law, who I love and by her own admission isn't a wordy or particularly demonstrative woman, lay on the floor behind me and just held me till it passed. Then I went to bed and got up to do it all again the next day.

I had spent hours and hours with the lawyers preparing, learning to be cross-examined, going over evidence and sometimes getting to admire the view across the whole harbour from the sixtieth floor. Stunning indeed and no doubt paid for by the $5000-a-day barrister charges. To be honest, he earned it and he was also generous about what he didn't charge for, like my solicitor who donated the last day of the proceedings on the grounds that it was a public flogging, in his words. Both lawyers were astounded by how the Coroner and police and other witnesses acted towards me. My solicitor said I was the most truthful witness he'd ever seen who was not believed. Those men were lovely to me.

By the time the inquest came around, my community support had gone. The friends of the last few years, with some notable exceptions, had vanished and to this day I do not know why. There was some gossip that I was drug addicted (I'm not and I wasn't) and I know that some women who had vindictive families and exes were scared to be associated with me as the Department of Community Services (DoCS) knew they knew me and marked their files accordingly.

Homebirthers were threatened fairly regularly across the country through these years and were scared to step out of line. Still, it was agonising when suddenly no one spoke to me, cared for my children, offered their friendship or sisterhood or were present for me through that tough time. The friends who were there for me will never be forgotten.

When I stepped outside on the first day of the inquiry while the other witnesses were cross-examined, I sat in the foyer of that low-ceilinged 1960s building on Parramatta Rd, opposite the Sydney University campus, closed my eyes and listened to harpsichords. Clutching the arms of the chair to keep myself from flying out the door, I was reminded of three years earlier when I clutched the arms of the chair in the custody sergeant's office as I was cautioned a few weeks after my stillbirth before I was questioned by detectives.

The court clerk called me and retrieved me from my seat near the door. It was a heart thumping moment as I walked in, went to the witness seat and was affirmed. It was noteworthy to me that those supporting me affirmed and those not supporting me, swore. I'm a lifelong atheist and could never swear on someone's religious text about truth. And then I was cross-examined for the first time of many over that week. I have mentioned earlier the ridiculous questions and assertions about my books, of which there are too many. I was calm, remembered my training and did not argue or pontificate. I am certain that Counsel Assisting expected me to be fired up and try to justify my political positions. I am sure they hoped to show me as a frothing crazy. I always disappoint on that score being surprisingly white, uptight and middle-class and even shaving my legs and wearing make-up for the event. I do sometimes wonder why I bothered since the perception was I am a two-headed neglectful mother regardless, but sometimes playing that game speaks to the optics the press convey.

It was hard. It was gruelling. There was assertion after assertion, which was a gaslighting misreading of everything I've ever done. As soon as the lawyer stopped and my barrister stood up and spoke gently to me, I cried. That's the thing when you're holding it all in through unkindness and then someone is kind so it all falls out. Did I want to stop for a break? No. I wanted to get it over with. Someone shoved the court tissue box at me, I poured my own water; we went on. Unsurprisingly, at the end of the day, the farcical jurisdiction hearing ended and the Coroner declared himself able to pass judgment on me. I had expected as much. No one would go through all that political posturing and then call it off. There was a woman to punish, after all.

Feminism on Trial

It was clear throughout that my feminism was on trial in this inquiry. My writings were scrutinised, my medical records from my son's birth were scrutinised (only my hospital records, though, not the actual record of care through the midwife I had at that time). My forums were used to apparently indicate that I encourage women to partake in risky behaviours and hide the consequences. I have found the continual insistence that I have hidden my stillbirth to be a bizarre assertion. I clearly did a very poor job of it since I was a front-page news story all over Australia[35] and even made it into newspapers in other parts of the world. I was accused of failing to grieve properly and thus being uncaring; more concerned with some birth experience than the babies. Shades of Lindy Chamberlain.[36] Women are always wrong.

My therapist wrote a letter which was given in evidence to the effect that Janet grieves normally and expresses deep sorrow and distress at her stillbirth. I was still monstrous in the eyes of the court. I was cross-examined about articles I'd written in 2004, a full five years prior to my stillbirth. I was cross-examined about things other people had written about me, without consulting me, and which weren't true. Those too were my fault. A social worker who was sent to attend me in the hospital had written that I had a sister called Val, who was an ambulance officer who attended the birth. In court, this was used as part of an argument to demonstrate my lack of credibility because it supposedly showed I was lying and covering up having had a freebirth. Except I hadn't covered that up at all but been completely frank with the doctors, nurses and midwives prior to my daughter's arrival who weren't particularly interested. The doctor who broke the news of her death to me actually said, "I'm terribly sorry, your baby has died of SIDS." To which I responded, gently, "Are you sure? I think she was stillborn …?"

I don't have a sister called Val. I don't have a sister who is an ambulance officer. And as a result I hadn't told the social worker any of this. Why she wrote it down is a complete mystery to me. Yet I was cross-examined about it and called a liar for denying it had occurred. She wasn't asked why she had put it in her notes. Likewise a journalist who was friends with a prominent obstetrician demanded he be allowed to give evidence because he'd interviewed me about birth politics. His sister is a midwife and he repeatedly emailed and telephoned me to say he feels a connection with me. I did not feel a connection with him and consider him to have stalked me. He stopped stalking me some years later.

My Big Lies

In order to demonstrate that the Coroner had jurisdiction over my baby's death, it had to be shown that she was born alive. I had said she was not born alive. The Coroner had said she was. Perhaps this is why it was so very difficult to get the jurisdiction hearing – which would have been an event without the media present. There are few rules to coronial inquiries – they take all kinds of evidence because they are fact-finding missions, not accusations. For some weeks into the eventual lead up to the event itself, my lawyers repeatedly asked for a jurisdiction hearing. Over and over we were told it wasn't possible. Eventually, Counsel Assisting agreed with the Coroner that it could run in tandem with the opening day of the inquest. It is difficult not to view this as a case of 'have-cake-and-eat-it-too', in a legal sense. It meant that everything would be discussed in the public eye, with full media attention. The likelihood that the Coroner himself would then decide he didn't have jurisdiction was vanishingly small. We had endured a number of unethical moments in the lead up to the inquiry – this was no different.

The Born Alive rule suggests that stillbirths are considered natural events and do not warrant the public scrutiny of an inquest. There are certainly times when this is utterly true. There are times it serves obstetrics too, such as the case of twins who died in utero in Melbourne because doctors injected the wrong foetus in a third trimester attempt to abort one foetus with potential health problems. After rushing to surgery, both babies were removed via caesarean section and declared dead. They were thus not Born Alive and no public inquiry required. The actions of the hospital staff clearly caused the death of both babies but since they died prior to the surgery to remove them from their mother's womb, no one could be publicly held accountable.[37] This rule is not applied so kindly in homebirth situations.

So the question of my daughter being alive at birth was not answered by the postmortem, which found she was already dead. Normally this would be enough to decide the matter but given the pursuit of me, it was not to be. Instead I was grilled on that first day about whether or not I had felt a pulse in her cord. Much emphasis was given to my knowledge of birthing matters but I maintained that I had not felt a cord pulse. But why, I was asked, did I say her cord *was* pulsing straight after the birth? The obstetrician's evidence indicated it was not uncommon for lay people, particularly in a heightened state which I was, holding my baby who wasn't breathing, to feel their own pulse echoed in something they touch which appeared to imply I might have been telling the truth, as he saw it. I was, of course, telling the truth but having said in that moment of life and death, "yes I believed her cord was pulsing" – because perhaps this was what I wanted to believe – they used this to justify the inquest into my birth. It feels cynical and cruel to exploit my vulnerability in that moment, but the whole exercise was both of those things so this would be no different. In the absence of scientific evidence that my baby breathed, normally the postmortem results would be used to decide such a question. But no: far better for them to use my own words and then deny me a change of mind. This was to prove my lack of credibility along with three other points.

One of the other Big Lies I was supposed to have told was that I'd had a short labour before transferring to hospital with my second baby. Actually I'd had a really long labour. I accept I lied about this. It harmed precisely no one and every single midwife and homebirthing woman in the courtroom knew why I'd told the staff this. I also explained clearly why I had said this and really, does it have any bearing whatsoever on a birth of a different child which then occurred three years later? You'd think not, but there you go.

When I discovered I was pregnant with my second child, we lived in Melbourne. By a strange quirk of fate, my partner was offered work in Sydney so we agreed he'd take it, we'd sell the house I adored in the northern suburbs, and head to Sydney. It was a rough process but luckily I had a somewhat easier pregnancy than my first. Our house was passed in at auction and despite the pressure from our real estate agents to accept a far lower price than they'd told us we should, I said we would hang on for a better offer. My partner went up to Sydney to begin his new job and I stayed in Melbourne to mother the toddler and grow the new babe.

After I'd felt hurt and unsatisfied in the care of my first midwife, I decided I would start a relationship with a new midwife in Sydney in an upfront way. I sought to impress upon her that I was keen for her emotional support and birth support, but retaining control over the decisions was deeply important to me since I did not feel this happened in my first birth and here I was with a scar to prove it.

This midwife is well regarded and lots of women know who she is because she told them I was her client when she was later justifying to people at large, why she dumped me from her care. I did not seek to publicise her name and even when I had heard details of my own experience via other women who'd heard it from her, I did not publicly write anywhere that she was my careprovider. I emailed asking her to please stop talking about me and adhere to my reasonable expectation of privacy which we should all be able to expect from anyone in healthcare. She had said to people that "Janet planned to freebirth all along," which pretty obviously wasn't true. I spent many hours writing my first birth story and answering her questions about my transfer. I knew she was a safe midwife to approach for a vaginal birth after a caesarean as she had a well-documented history of supporting women in normal birth that hospitals would not support. A good sign, I thought. She was also my sister's midwife at the time and my sister was pleased with her care. Time passed in Melbourne and despite me saying I wished we could have more phone time getting to know one another, and her not calling me, I thought it would work out once I got to Sydney. Maybe she's not a phone person?

I got to Sydney and began appointments with her. By this point I was at the end of my pregnancy and around that time, women go to weekly appointments. She came to our house, used the Doppler on my belly (which didn't thrill me but I was prepared to compromise since she hadn't seen me all pregnancy), and I worked on building rapport. She was pleasant but a little distant. One night I woke up from a dream imagining that I was in labour to find what looked like a pool of blood in the bed. I rang her and asked her to come over because I wanted some reassurance and the kind of loving care midwives give women. I also called my friend in Queensland who flew down immediately and I spent some time thinking maybe the birth was near.

The midwife declared it a hindwater leak[38] and my friend generously said she was glad of the dress rehearsal. The midwife listened to babe, who was fine. Took my blood pressure, which was always fine. The days progressed. The leak sealed, as they do, and about a week later at my appointment the midwife said, "You have a really big baby in there, already over 4kg. I think you're going to need another caesarean. I'm happy to refer you to someone else if you think I'm too negative to be in your birth space." Then she finished my appointment by taking my blood pressure, which was now sky high. I said, "Thank you, please send me some names if you feel this way," and I politely showed her to her car, remembering to thank her for the care she'd shown my sister. I came back inside and had the second panic attack of my life.

My first birth ended in surgery, which I realised in retrospect I did not need. I felt abandoned by my midwife whose postpartum care was nothing short of shoddy. With my second birth I had placed my trust in another careprovider and here she was dumping me. Cue me vomiting into the sink and swearing there was NO

WAY I was going to hospital. My partner, for whom freebirth had not felt like a good option, agreed that freebirth was the best option at this point. I was hoping the midwife would do as she suggested, but she never sent me any contacts. I rang a doula who lived several hours away and who I'd met briefly the week before. I knew she had a history of picking up after midwives who failed their clients. I asked her if I went into labour would she come and she said yes. As I awaited email contacts from the main midwife, I managed to eat some dinner having stopped vomiting and I went to bed. And here came labour. I woke up in the morning in labour. I am sure the panic attack facilitated that. We were otherwise completely healthy as time showed.

The beautiful doula came and she stayed the two nights and days it took to birth that babe. She never asked for money, in fact, she refused it. There are women in birth who really do it for the women; she was one. At the end of the very long birth, 60 hours roughly, I eventually climbed out of the pool with the baby and lay exhausted on the futon in my study. I started to bleed. First my partner rang around the local midwives, including the one who'd dumped me, who he rang first. No one came, most didn't answer the call, only one returned the call a few days later. After my previous hospital experience, I was inclined to go earlier rather than later as advocating for motherbaby once the baby is born is very different from advocating while you still have the baby safely inside you. Partner rang an ambulance, I ate some raw placenta which basically stopped the bleeding by the time they arrived. Nevertheless, I felt in my state of pure exhaustion that it would be better to be safe, go to the hospital and have some Syntocinon (an artificial form of oxytocin) to completely stop the post partum bleeding. So I went in the ambulance.

When I arrived at the hospital I planned not to tell them I'd had a freebirth because I was concerned about child protection. We may have been fine, which we were, but everyone in the birth world knows all it takes is a staff member who hates homebirth to report a woman and there's big trouble for her family. We all knew women and midwives who'd experienced it and I didn't want it for my family. I said I'd had a very short labour and the midwife didn't make it so I was here for some help now, please. They asked who the midwife was and I didn't tell them. I did not want a hospital knowing she'd 'withdrawn her care' from a woman so imminently close to birth in case some other staff member thought this was a reasonable excuse to report her. I wanted to protect my family and I wanted to protect a midwife, even one who'd hurt me deeply and would hurt me much more deeply over the coming years.

So I got the Syntocinon infusion and then they stitched me up (badly), said a few silly things, and a lot of people came in to 'look at the homebirth' which was pretty bizarre. One was a New Zealand midwife who said homebirth was pretty normal where she lived so, "Good on you." Babe was checked, briefly out of my arms, and was of course perfectly bonny. The midwives gave me poor breastfeeding advice which made me laugh since I was still breastfeeding the toddler at home from time to time and had no trouble breastfeeding. The babe was a natural. We went home more tired than I have ever been. I sat in the loungeroom in the dark of night finally able to marvel over this amazing being I'd made and birthed right over there in a deflating birth pool. I couldn't lift my toddler after the blood loss and long, long birth but I could snuggle him plenty.

So here in court we are told another example of my terrible ways, all these years later. The midwife who'd dumped me kept all the emails we'd exchanged and sent them to the police. I had given her detailed descriptions of what was most important to me in the event of another hospital transfer. I had repeatedly discussed transferring with her. What did she say in her police statement? She was concerned I would refuse to transfer and she believed I had been too unwell to birth at home that time since my blood pressure was very high. Had it previously been high? No. Was it high when she'd 'withdrawn her care'? Why, yes, it was. And is that any wonder? The Crown decided she would be their key midwifery witness and she was given my statements and my birth video to watch. This was just another cruel blow and loss of privacy. Someone who had denied me care to justify her own unethical actions called to provide 'unbiased' evidence about me? How would that work? In the end, my barrister was able to have her removed and another midwife brought in with whom I had no pre-existing relationship. Was it better? Well, yes. But still the loss of privacy was distressing.

Yet another Big Lie by me would have been funny under other circumstances but was kind of tragically silly. I would dearly love to speak to the social worker who caused it all but what would

I say to her? Take better notes? After I was left in the hospital room alone, my supportive friend having been taken away for questioning by police, the standard on-call social worker was assigned to me. I've experienced such folks before and largely found them well meaning but not especially helpful. But I know it can be useful to get the traumatic event out of your head as soon as possible and begin processing so I thought I would do that. And as I had on other hospital occasions, I assumed staff are there to help. I told her the story of my birth, I told her I ran a homebirth group, I told her my friend had attended my birth. I rambled on about not having slept and mentioned something about this friend from Queensland being the daughter of an ambulance officer. This isn't why she was at my births, she was there because I loved her dearly and we were very close despite our geographical distance. So the social worker wrote down that Janet runs a 'human birth group', which really made me wonder what other kinds of birth groups there are? And she wrote that I told her my sister, Val, attended my birth and is an ambulance officer.

I did not say this.

Counsel Assisting said I had told the social worker I had an ambulance officer present in order to make it seem like I hadn't freebirthed. She pushed and pushed the idea that I had hidden my freebirth from everyone. I had not. I was open with the staff at the hospital that I had had a freebirth. No one judged me or spoke unkindly to me. I was well treated as a patient, overall. I did not tell the social worker then, with a view to somehow cover up everything I'd already said to the medical staff, that I'd had an ambulance officer present, much less my sister Val, the ambulance officer. I do have a sister. She's not called Val and she doesn't drive ambulances. None of that mattered; it was chalked up as another of my character failings: another Big Lie.

Questioning me on notes taken by other people seemed a peculiar way to get to the truth. Why was the social worker not called and asked to explain her notes? How could I be responsible for what someone else had written down? Hospital staff sometimes write notes hours later when the emergency has passed. We all know this. The note taking system is not as infallible as people believe and this too is well known in medical circles. People are only human and sometimes notes will be inaccurate. This was some major inaccuracy though and really did me no favours. I should like to ask her to be more careful next time so her notes won't be used to condemn a grieving mother.

The last part of undermining my credibility was to misinterpret my feelings around my first birthing experience. After my son was born and I flailed desperately seeking support but finding little, I delved more into the writings of Leilah McCracken. It is she who probably coined the term, 'birthrape', which people find so objectionable.[39] I wrote about my experience in the hospital system with the obstetrician who did not remove her hand from my vagina while I breathlessly tried to tell her to stop and beetled up the bed on my back away from her. This moment haunted me in the months and years after my surgery and I even dreamt about it. This was rape. If rape is a person refusing to remove themselves from your body after entering it, it was a rape. If she had put her hand in my vagina in the carpark and I'd asked her to stop, it would be assault. Somehow, despite what I thought was clear about this incident, Counsel Assisting insisted I said my caesarean surgery was a rape. I didn't. I'd never said this because it wasn't. Personally I was clear that yes, for what it's worth, I had shakily signed that consent form, though my barely recognisable signature would bring me to tears when I saw it. But my discussion of the vaginal exam to which I withdrew my consent, and consider an assault, was laid over the top of my distaste for the surgery and made into a gotcha moment. It was manipulated to say, here is your signature, therefore the surgery was not a rape. This was then a lie which went to deny any credibility I may have had. Except I never said it since I don't perceive the surgery to have been a rape. It is hard to imagine lawyers cannot tell the difference between a description of one event, in the course of another, and see a discrete event being labelled an assault but not the overall event to which it led. Perhaps the term 'birthrape' was a confusing one and they interpreted it in this way. Obviously they could have sought clarity on this but didn't since the narrative that I was a liar was vital to setting up an inquest.

No End in Sight

It had previously been decided that with Easter approaching (the final day of that week was Good Friday), the inquest would be limited to the four days Monday to Thursday. There was some sage muttering about taxpayer money (another reason given for not allowing me a jurisdiction hearing) and agreement from Counsel Assisting. It didn't turn out like that but I had really hoped I might be out of that hell by Thursday – while still having the agonising wait until the findings were released.

The following days are a bit of a blur. There was more news footage, the cameras had chased us down the road to lunch on the first day, though a friend tried to shield me by walking in front. I forgot to change into my sunglasses and had to wander down the road in indoor glasses, which didn't feel very protective. Every day, my barrister would ask for a recess and we'd step into the legal team breakout rooms and he'd say the Coroner and Counsel Assisting were acting unethically again, and I could go to the Supreme Court and, in his opinion, win the call. And I'd ask what would happen then, to which he'd respond that they'd reschedule the inquest. I could not bear the thought of stringing it out any longer since I'd realised as soon as the idea of another inquest was raised that it would happen and more years and money were not what I wanted (or could afford). So we went back in.

My father attended a couple of days, which was surprising to me. You will remember he had taken me home from the hospital after my daughter was born but he was a man with few skills at intimacy who had rarely been a supportive parent. My mother died in 2002 before I'd had children and given that she too had had a pregnancy loss, I was almost glad she was not there to be triggered mightily by these proceedings. My father was always a stalwart, somewhat emotionally austere person. But he was a great raconteur and bon vivant with his friends rather than his family. From early on after the birth he had said to me repeatedly that he did not understand why 'they' were going after me at all. I had a few stabs at explaining that uppity women, feminist mothers, women who oppose the obstetric monopoly, don't make friends with powerful people, but he could not take it on board. While a keen and committed bohemian Leftie, he could not envision a way to apply those critiques to women's lives beyond the obvious points of equal pay or condemnation of sexual harassment, I took to nodding and agreeing what a mystery it was. The second last day of the inquest, he suddenly began to cry in the breakout room which stopped the lawyers in their tracks and me too. He kept stammering "poor mummy" over and over which I think meant he was overwhelmed. Was he overwhelmed by his memories of being a father experiencing loss? By relief that Mum wasn't there to see me pilloried? I don't know. I doubt he could have articulated it and he's not around to ask now since he died in late 2016. I miss him.

On the afternoon of the second last day, my lawyers were prepared for summing up the following day and my barrister announced this in court. Nodding all round. I had also been told that I would be allowed to give a statement on the last day so I had been busily constructing that in my head all week. We turned up in court the following morning and Counsel Assisting and the Coroner had changed their minds and a new day for summing up was organised, in the months ahead. My lawyers were not pleased. That's two extra days which they now needed to find in their calendars: one for summing up and one for handing down the findings. My barrister simply couldn't do it because he would be appearing at a murder trial at the next scheduled dates. In the end my solicitor appeared for me at those final two days.

I did, however, still get to deliver my statement to the inquiry on the last day of the hearings in Glebe. As the parent of the babe I was permitted to offer a statement to the court once my evidence was concluded, reflecting on the loss of my daughter in my life, and that of her family. The statement was tendered as evidence.

My Statement to the Court

Thank you for the opportunity to address the court. Firstly, I would like to thank his Honour for the words of sympathy he extended to my family yesterday. I found it a moment of kindness and humanity in what has been a foreign experience to us and I am grateful for his genuine acknowledgement of our loss.

When a woman is pregnant, it is a family and a community who expects a baby. Roisin has a brother and sister who anticipated her arrival with all the uncomplicated joy of young children. They were five and almost three at the time of her birth. Roisin has grandparents, Trevor's parents and my father, as my mother is deceased and never met any of my children. She has aunts, uncles and cousins who also awaited her arrival with joy. She has a father who first held her at birth as he did his previous daughter and son. She has a mother who only held a moving babe in her belly, not in her arms. I am a mother of three children with only two visible to the world in which we move.

Had my birth ended differently and we were not in this court, I could share the life and joys of my three-year-old daughter. I could share the interactions she would have had with her siblings. Her father could report on his relationship with her – shoulder rides and pretend disappearing games were popular with her siblings and I can only imagine so it may have been for Roisin.

Since I cannot share these, I can perhaps share instead some of the meaning of her loss to me, and to her family. The loss of a babe is a visceral, primal wound. It is a loss of such magnitude that it echoes through our close community of friends, many of whom have attended this week, who held us in love then and now. Her loss will form a part of my family's tapestry for generations as has the stillbirth of my nephew and my mother's loss of my younger brother.

The loss of this child to me as her mother has also changed me in profound ways. I had hoped to call this daughter Carys, which means love in Welsh. Her father named her as we were in the hospital, and chose a beautiful Irish name to reflect my family's heritage. What Roisin has come to mean in my life is an awakening to love and to compassion, and perhaps it is fitting her name means rose since I hope to always grow in love as a tribute to her. This child will never grace family occasions with her presence; she will forever remain a newborn even when I am a woman of eighty. I will feel her loss every day for the rest of my life.

My older daughter has now lived more than half her life as we have awaited these proceedings. My son tells me now, "When the inquest is over, mummy, let's never talk about it again, please." This inquiry has cast a long shadow through these last three years. I hope the court will forgive me for commenting that it can also be an onerous process on top of such a loss as we have experienced. Despite this I am grateful I live in a country where the unexpected loss of a baby is recognised as worthy of community attention and I hope these proceedings offer hope and information which help other bereaved families or help those hoping to reduce stillbirths in Australia.

Our loss has touched another family deeply as well and I can only offer such a small thank you in the face of the generosity, love and care given freely by Alyson (a pseudonym) and her own family. I have no other words with which to express my deep gratitude to her but I hope she knows I will feel indebted to her for the rest of my life. There are so many other friends who I will not name but I hope I have at some point, or will at some point, communicate my deepest thanks to each of you and your families.

My barrister and my solicitor have cared for us through this last while in a way which offers a small glimpse into the hearts of two very special and dedicated men. Again, a debt of gratitude which can never be repaid but one which I hope I can communicate to them in some small way much dwarfed by their own compassionate response to us in a time of stress.

While it is I who have written these words, and delivered them, I cannot leave Roisin's father out of this narrative as he has been so frequently disappeared from media and other reports of the loss of his own child. He is a father to a babe he will never see grow up and two living children whom he cherishes deeply. Despite our separation last year, I know him to be an honourable, loving man with a deep commitment to family and hope he always remembers the love we shared as I know he will always carry in his heart the pain of the lost child for whom we both wished so dearly.

No words can ever do justice to the experience of losing a child. All we can do is form small sentences which go almost nowhere to touch the distress, the grief, the yearning, the slow turning pain. I feel grateful that I have been allowed to say some of these important things which live in the confines of my mind, my home, my family and my community but which are necessarily invisible to those more removed from our sphere. Thank you.

~

I never approach Easter without feeling the shadow of these four days in court. When Easter is a long way from Roisin's birth date, it simply stretches that ongoing and unrelenting unease of March and April. When Easter is close to her birthday, it is like revisiting that time. Exhaustion does not come close to describing what it was like. I had little children, I was a single mother by then, and I had the children with me for that week. They still talk about how wonderful that Easter was because I stocked up on chocolate and bought them a new movie on DVD and we basically ate chocolate and I lay down as much as possible. It was an absolute marathon during those years and I still had submissions and then findings to come. Pacing myself wasn't really an option but managing day to day simply had to be.

Submissions

For submissions in early winter, the inquest was moved from the old premises in Glebe out to the new court complex in Parramatta, where criminal matters are normally heard. It was a sunny June day. After the four days of the inquest before Easter, I had walked in front of the bathroom mirror one night and taken scissors to my medium length hair to avoid being recognised in the street which was happening a bit. It's funny what people 'see' and that simply cutting off my hair to a bob made me unrecognisable. I did not want people approaching me in the street when I was out with my small children. In the end the media didn't come looking for me that day; they just replayed old Glebe footage of me walking down the street amongst the scrum trying to not trip over. And they came up with the headlines a few days later for the findings like, "Baby's death due to rash mother, says irate coroner."[40]

To be frank, my patience with judgment being passed over me in every way was about done. I listened to the list of points condemning me as the worst mother since Lindy Chamberlain, slid down to my shoulder blades in the seat and studied the laces on my boots. Counsel Assisting began the litany of my misdemeanours dating back to 2003 when I was apparently already a bad mother. It continued in that vein through the various deliberate misreadings of my character and actions to the present including things I had written since the initial hearing.

My solicitor stood up. By his own admission, he's a solicitor because he's not that keen on the adversarial chat but he is good at it whatever he thinks. Following their lead, he also began in 2003. Immediately he was stopped as this was deemed not relevant. It set the tone for the day. Despite intense frustration on his part he was pretty much unable to present anything resembling my views, my side, my experience, my voice, anything. Every point was shot down by Counsel Assisting or the Coroner on the grounds of relevance or my supposed taste for lying. He bought me lunch and apologised for the public flogging I'd received. I hugged him and said at least it's almost over.

During the initial four days of the inquest I had a profound sense of acceptance and surrender and also of forgiveness as I sat in court with assumptions, anger, misinformation and untruths being paraded and somehow associated with me. I felt that in order to put a woman and her family who've lost a baby through three years of uncertainty, dubious legal workings and punishment, you have to be really disconnected from your humanity and deeply invested in the oppression of women. I saw intense undisguised anger from lawyers who should be without prejudice in a courtroom. I saw judgment from police officers and ambulance officers. But, as I sat in the stand being cross-examined, and then in my seat during submissions, my overwhelming sense was of compassion for such hardness of heart. Listening to yourself being misinterpreted and perceived as evil is a trial but it can be borne. It ends even though the memories linger. Those living with such disconnection from their heart may well be on a lifelong journey removed from love. That is really sad.

Chapter Six

The Findings

After we were done with submissions, now to the findings. I had said to my lawyers at the start of the inquest that the findings would be that I am a neglectful, dangerous mother with outrageous beliefs who practically killed my baby who would definitely, without a doubt, have lived if she'd been born in a hospital. There could be no other findings. It was also important to my emotional health to note again at this time that the Coroner had refused, despite my barrister petitioning for such, to give me a guarantee of exemption from prosecution. I was thus aware that arresting me had never been ruled out. Whatever the reasons had been for why the inquest suddenly could have another day on the taxpayer, I couldn't help feeling it likely that one of those reasons was Counsel Assisting wanting to go through all evidence with a fine toothcomb to see if I could be charged.

I was especially disturbed in retrospect by this decision a few years later when a man who'd been charged with (but found not guilty of) murdering his partner was granted immunity from prosecution in order to have his testimony heard at a coronial inquiry trying to find what had happened to the murdered man. Knowing there was a receipt for a shovel and CCTV footage showing the men leaving a venue together, and that Ockham's Razor would rather indicate one man murdered the other, he was allowed to step up and name where his lover was buried and not face any legal consequences.[41] I am sadly relieved for the victim's family who were then able to reclaim his body. I confess it was a somewhat lip-pursing moment for me to see a highly probable murderer given that kind of legal privilege when a mother of a stillborn baby was not.

So while I knew in my head that if the Coroner, police or Counsel Assisting had thought at any point in the proceedings I should be charged, they would have closed down the inquest immediately and done so, I nevertheless still lived with lingering fears and uncertainty. By this point, as mentioned earlier, the kids and I had lost many in our local community. I knew the media would be stirring up more hatred towards me. I took the kids and we stayed in a hotel the night before the findings were handed down so the police would at least have to look for me to arrest me. But we had decided not to go to court and hear the findings. My solicitor attended on 28 June 2012 in order to argue on my behalf that my birth video should not be released to the TV channels who wanted it. They already had a recording of the Triple 000 call my baby's distraught father had made. One of the channels used footage of a friend's homebirth to run their story. We call her my body double now.

I think those things often backfire for the media though. They are trying to massage our thinking and manufacture our consent to the supposedly awfully dangerous crime of birthing at home. The words are all about risk but the images are of a woman birthing in her own space, respected and held by those who love her. In a world filled with notions of birth as dangerous and diabolical for birthing women, I think these images do something quite unintended and show women that birth can be under their control and performed with love.

And so to the findings. After the Coroner had brought the findings down, my solicitor phoned me in the hotel I had stayed overnight. "Are the findings what we expected?" I asked him, and the answer was that indeed they were. Later, when I got a copy of the findings, I saw that the first page of the document by the Deputy State Coroner says Janet Fraser is a possible leader in a movement called Joyous Birth. I stopped reading. It's clear that if a document opens with something so patently, demonstrably untrue, nothing good is going to come after that. I think part of it was simply the complete lack of internet literacy of that Coroner. He truly had no idea what was a forum, a blog, Facebook or anything else. I didn't, and don't, run a movement. I did, and do, own a website called Joyous Birth. As we had pointed out in court, there was not at the time of my stillbirth an Australian parenting forum which didn't have a homebirth or even a freebirth section. Were they also running movements and corrupting minds? But it was obviously necessary to paint me as crazed and dangerous as possible, otherwise why spend all that money and time condemning me? If I were just a mother, at home, with a computer, encouraging other women to learn about birth, breastfeeding and human rights, it might not be nearly so impressive – and so bad.

The findings continued with the statement by the Coroner that it was my socio-political beliefs that led to the death of my baby – which could be read on my website. As to the cause of her death, it was found that my daughter had *likely* (my emphasis) stopped breathing as a result of a 'hypoxic episode' [not enough oxygen] *after the umbilical cord became tangled around her neck.*

Surely, as I gave birth to my baby I would have noticed any cord entanglement around her neck but there was none. And even if I hadn't noticed, surely my partner would have seen it as well as my friend? In fact we had photographic and video evidence that this was not the case.

As for the Coroner's comment that lack of oxygen had *likely* lead to my baby's death – another unproven assumption as neither the postmortem nor any other observations from ambulance officers and hospital personnel could 'prove' why my daughter had died.

In sum, the findings consisted of unproven assumptions of what *might* have been the reason for my baby's death. The overarching message of the findings – apart from a strong damnation of my beliefs as expressed on the Joyous Birth website – was that had this baby been born in a hospital she would have lived – another unproven assumption.

Often after an inquest, recommendations are provided to avoid such situations in future. This usually involves relevant public authorities attending, such as a representative of the police if a matter involves a police investigation and evidence like a death in custody or a missing person's case. WorkSafe might attend if a death has occurred in a workplace and they're seeking to learn how another might be avoided. The Coroner's findings after the inquest into my daughter's death included no recommendations.

The NSW Health Department, despite having had a say in the questions posed to commence the inquest – that is, asking if I posed a danger to public health – were not required to implement any recommendations. The question the Health Department posed wasn't really answered since how could it be? Where was the demonstrable link between my writing and an increase in women birthing at home with or without midwives? Earlier during the pre-Easter inquest, the Coroner had announced in the courtroom, with me present, words to the effect that there was no point offering recommendations because women like me swim so far outside the flags that no warnings would be heeded. Yet now that the findings did indeed not include any recommendations, what did that mean? Either my work is a danger or it's not.

Given that the entire inquest was examining what is essentially a deeply unfortunate but often unavoidable event occurring around six times a day in Australia – the birth of a stillborn baby – describing women who birth at home as a danger to ourselves and our babies doesn't prevent stillbirth. Describing hospital birthing women as responsible mothers doesn't prevent stillbirth either.

It was a stark moment when the point of the whole debacle became abundantly clear to me: the outcome of the inquest was to frighten women and punish me. The excuse that women like me pay no attention to warnings so why issue any, is clearly ridiculous. The reality, of course, is that everyone knew it was a farce but it was a farce with the cherry on top of punishing a woman who encourages autonomy in other women.

Tellingly, to the best of my knowledge, I am the only Australian freebirthing woman whose stillbirth warranted an inquest. I know of a couple of other women who had stillbirths at home without obstetric attendants. The police investigation eventually decided 'natural causes' were to blame and thus an inquest was unnecessary. Those women still went through the invasion of their spaces at home and confiscation of computers and cameras, but at least their names weren't made public and no other action was taken. It is hard to avoid the conclusion that it was my outspokenness in the face of medico-legal authorities which led to my very public condemnation.

Considering I have never advocated women seek anything other than what is available to us by law – the right to decide how, where, and with whom we birth – and that I have exhorted medical communities to abide by the law, this seems peculiar. If our patriarchal society thinks however, that women are public property, that the foetus must be protected from us at all costs and that mothers are least invested in the survival of our offspring, perhaps then it all makes sense.

Just thinking back to those days and weeks before, during and after the inquest to the day of the findings brings me to the point of feeling nauseous. My children and I left the hotel and went home during the day the findings were released after my solicitor had called me. He told me that he'd successfully argued the video of my birth not be given to the television stations. It is worth noting that unfortunately this kept *my* version of events away from the media: even the most hostile witnesses agreed that the video showed a perfectly normal birth followed by the commencement of CPR. And the medical people agreed that CPR was performed normally. But I did not want my naked body on the news all over the country.

Another point that upset me greatly was that while it was unnecessary to release the name of my baby, the Coroner said early on it was in the public interest. Is there any public interest served other than to make my baby, who never breathed, more of a living baby in the eyes of the public? And me and my views on birthing more of a Bad Mother? If it had been 'The Mother and The Baby' throughout the coverage, the benefit of the state about scaring women out of home or freebirths would have been diminished. In theory, despite the Coroner naming me and my baby, media are not supposed to identify people in a way which may cause their other children to be identified. By naming us both, it showed my living children did not matter in the eyes of the court. My children all mean love to me though my missing baby is only love since I have no living form of her. To hear her name from the mouths of those who seek to exploit her death causes immense pain.

The day after

Shrinking my life from a symphony
endowed with nuance, shade, light, melody
and counterpoint plus harmonics.
Reducing me to a parody unrecognisable.
A bitter cacophony.
Do you realise how your clever hatreds form
naught but the accompaniment to your woman-hating dirge?
Each aria says to every woman,
that she is lesser.
Even if she doesn't realise it yet,
and still believes she is free.
She is a vessel of evil.
Fit only for incubator status.
Everything defective from skin to frame to thoughts.
Shrinking my loss, my baby, the grief to dot points.
Obliterating humanity.
Enabling hatred.
How did we move so far from love
that a mother's grief became the vehicle
with which to punish her?

The night following the release of the findings was a peak time for hate mail and death threats. The purpose of the findings was to make sure the world knew I was a bad mother whose child had died a preventable death due to my own weird belief systems and recalcitrant behaviour. It worked. The dirty dealings, the politics, the lies and the wider context of how we hate women in Australia ceases to exist once a 'definitive' version of events is presented in court.

When the media's favourite cherry-picked condemnations from the findings of me hit the news, the hate mail started rolling in. Once I noticed it, I called a friend and she dealt with it. She put a forward on my email for words like death, die, murder, murderer, bullet, bitch, hanging and the like. She contacted my local police station and informed them I was receiving death threats regularly. "Print them out and attend the station" was the response. I'm unsure how you might trace an electronic communication without having the whole electronic thread but it was clear the local police were not going to do anything about these threats. They had, after all, been part of the three ambulances, five cop cars and a forensic vehicle called to my home from our "baby not breathing" Triple 000 call.

I still got the 'polite' emails that simply called me crazy, unhinged or satanic and I disposed of those myself with a quick swipe. I didn't have to read anything but the first line. As someone once said to me, you don't need to drink the whole bath to know it's bath water you're drinking. One line is sufficient.

The phone rang and it was a friend telling me that a notorious North American blogger had published my full address on her blog along with the alleged findings which were, as yet, still unavailable to the public. I had to wonder about her sources and what it is to live in a valley of hatreds. But I didn't wonder for too long because it was just plain unpleasant to contemplate. Obviously her concern for my daughter didn't extend to the safety of my earthside children. I could not fathom this kind of behaviour; it was so very alien to me. Apart from being upsetting, it was a clear sign that we live in sad times where this kind of behaviour is acceptable to someone who claims to be a healer of the sick. Since it was overseas, Australian law and the publication suppression order on my home address did not apply. Even though she eventually agreed to my lawyer's polite request to redact my address (it was later removed from the site), it's out there now, the cat is out of the bag and it's on other blogs and never to be private again. I never call her by name because I don't like to dignify hatred with a response. But I hope it gave her readers pause that she was prepared to endanger me and my other children despite claiming to care for my dead baby. This American blogger, who has devoted most of her writing life to attacking women who birth at home and breastfeed, was used as a news source in Australia through my years of dealing with police, media and the Crown Solicitors.

My children and I lived in the home where my children were born. Like others of its vintage, it has a front verandah and the windows of the two front facing bedrooms are directly accessible from the front yard. I was not sure if some of the "you're-nothing-a-bullet-wouldn't-fix" crew might act on that after the American blogger published my address. For a week we slept on the couch which was in the next room past those bedrooms so there was an extra layer of house for a Molotov cocktail to burn through.

I had already received lots of hate mail at the time my baby was born. Probably more than I received after the inquest. Perhaps the three years of the legal process wore some people down and they lost interest. Perhaps some of them had second thoughts about abusing a woman who had lost a baby. I hope so, for it would probably speak to their growth and humanity. Sometimes the hate mail was anonymous, sometimes it was signed in full. It was fairly equally spread between those claiming to be men or women. There were healthcare workers who occasionally wrote to tell me how sorry they were for my loss and that they see stillbirths relatively often, which judging from the perinatal data, is true. There are approximately six stillbirths a day in Australia, after all, and more than 99% of them occur in hospitals. Stillbirth is no respecter of venue or cast, which is something all birth workers know despite the constant waving of the dead baby card as a way to control homebirthing or freebirthing women.[42]

I still get hate mail these days. I sometimes post about it on Facebook because I feel like I need to acknowledge it, but I don't read it very often. I don't read any of the media, open letters or blog entries, which claim to be about me or addressed to me. It is not about me, it's a reflection of the person who wrote it. So when I get emails from people who claim to loathe me, I feel sad for the anger and hatred they carry. I know that many of the women who write about me are carrying unaddressed, unacknowledged, untreated trauma from obstetrics and other forms of violence against women. You can't live your life without experiencing it in some form. I know that many of the fathers who write to me are carrying the pain and fear of witnessing what their partners have experienced and that they really want that to have been for a good reason since they felt helpless in the face of it – which they were. I know that our society breathes and eats cognitive dissonance or it just wouldn't look like it does. So many people are confused, unable to see past what the propaganda tells them and in pain from the effort of twisting themselves into what they think they ought to be.

I fully realise the irony that more hate mail will appear in response to me writing this book. So in case you missed it, this is what I think of your hate mail: I'm sorry you have so little compassion for self and others. I'm sorry your life has such hatred in it. I hope that you move towards love and find ways to be in the world which are nurturing for you and those around you. I wish you love.

I realise that birth, death, women's rights and feminism are some of the hottest buttons in western society. Mixing them up is a potent cocktail which rushes to some people's heads and leads to some big reactions. The misogyny on which our society is based lives in all of us, some of us just feel more free to let it out and share it, especially towards women we perceive as transgressive, like me.

Conclusion

I lived for some years with the fear of losing my children, about whom there were Department of Community Services reports, and the fear of prison. I found myself asking my, by then dead, mother for help. Please, Mum, don't let them take me away from the kids. I had bought some bed linen a few years previously because it reminded me of my favourite 1960s linen from my childhood. It was cream with little pink roses on one side and stripes on the other. My mind somehow latched onto prison linen having stripes and I could never bear to have that side showing. It wasn't rational but in a world so irrational that babies die and children have to face the potential loss of their mother, it became a bit of a talisman. A couple of years ago, I gave those sheets and pillow slips away to another single mother who could use them without always being reminded of fearful events.

There's some research on emergency workers which indicates that while post-traumatic stress is high in the group, so are indications of post-traumatic growth. The hypothesis is that this is because they can make meaning of the trauma and grow and learn from it. It's considered 'coherent', that is, you can make a new narrative of improved knowledge from the trauma, not only feel lost and victimised.

I relate to this partly through a feminist lens and partly through a Zen lens. I understand much of what I've been put through has been done to me because of my status as a woman, mother and public feminist. So it feels less like being picked on individually. I feel similarly about the instances of personal trauma inflicted by individuals: this only happens because I live in a patriarchal society not because I'm internally flawed. The Zen has a similarly depersonalising action in my life. Basically I'm pretty unimportant and my griefs are only as large as me, which is bloody insignificant in the whole universe.

This doesn't mean I haven't unpacked my contributions to situations in which I've found myself, a process in which therapy was a blessing. I also think that feminism gives us a way to take action which is why so many of us work in birth, work with women escaping violent men and with other groups supporting women. We use our experiences to fuel that passion and we make meaning of our pain by using that knowledge to help other women. The personal is political, it's true. And the political is very personal.

It's all a delicate dance but I want to offer some hope that's based in reality and not just wishing darkness away or pretending it didn't happen or internalising it and making it all our fault. Once all the furore dies down we are left with the wreckage of our lives, making meaning from the trauma inflicted, and our surviving that trauma. I used my first childbirth trauma to create a space for women so I would never again hear a woman say, "I wish I knew I could do it differently." I wanted women to know there were alternatives to the mainstream obstetric machine, which does not value motherbaby.

Last year was a decade since my stillbirth and I'm writing this in the following year, in the month which brings me undone. The year before I asked women to come to my home that day. Some women I don't know very well but who live locally came and there was quite a buzz of talk, that beautiful sound of women's voices. Other friends stayed late into the night when I finally let go and wept. Going home the night after my birth, with no baby, to a home covered with the evidence of police searching and the profound loss of privacy which only increased over time, is still held within me. The memories of the following week of a postmortem performed without my consent, avoiding the news, supporting my children, still flow through me.

We talk about triggers a lot nowadays but *life* is the trigger and it is up to me to manage it. I have learnt that love is the only act which matters in life. I have learnt that we stray from it at our peril. I have learnt what it is to be truly alone and what it is to have a heart that flies open easily and tears that spring forth at the least provocation. I have become used to having to steady myself on stage when I speak about issues that matter because grief this large can never be contained and it finds a way through the human frame no matter where or what you're doing. My baby meant love, to me. To have her sullied by scalpels of steel and print is to have my soul irreparably carved into. I cannot imagine how it might be to grieve to a timetable of one's own making. To have it ebb and flow as you age, as other children grow but those milestones never happen with the babe that died. To never have to wonder if now is the moment I need to tell someone to google my name and then let them decide if they still want to be seen with me. I let the machine roll over me so my other children would have a mother in their lives.

I always give this advice to women going through horrible events, particularly courtroom things: it will end. You don't know when, but one way or another, it will end. You won't die. You will sometimes want the process to kill you so you don't have to live with it any more, but it will not. You will live through it. Because that's what happened to me. The processes end, but the pain they caused does not and probably never will.

Advocating for women means advocating for all 'choices' not just the ones you'd make or the ones which suit your politics. They mean I also advocate for women who 'choose' booked surgeries despite the known risks to women and babies of such actions. I am from a feminist school which does not recognise the power of 'choice' as above all else, and as if it were free of social influence. I do not suggest a model of birth where we present all the options as equal because some are patently not the normal way for humans to be born. There is no moral judgment in saying this. It is, quite simply, a fact.

Humans have evolved to birth, and be birthed, which makes it simply the *normal* start to life earthside. It is both a special and unremarkable bodily process in a similar way our beating hearts or our breathing are special yet unexceptional processes. Birth is made meaningful by our interpretation of it as a spiritual journey but, sadly, as is more common nowadays, as a terrifying journey of unparalleled risk. We have made it other than normal because we have normalised the male body in all ways and thus childbirth, only performed by women, is going to stand outside of what is normal. It has already been pathologised beyond all recognition to a point where major abdominal surgery – a caesarean – is considered not on a par but *superior* to normal birth.

Reframing our births to use our own names for them is too shocking a step for obstetrics. I was criticised in the inquest for having written about my own birth as just a birth, suggesting that birthing after previous surgery might just be called a birth rather than a pathologising term: trial of scar, trial of labour, or even the well meant VBAC, vaginal birth after caesarean. This is the triumph of the surgeons and their system. I have long said obstetrics falls in the nexus between misogyny and profit. I stand by that. Bearing in mind however that booked caesareans are supported and promoted by obstetricians and television producers alike, and the 'right to choose' surgery is never under threat, I'm comfortable advocating for women's autonomy to birth normally.

We know from countless studies that most women want a normal, physiological birth. They want to achieve this supposedly normal birth in a hospital setting and they believe it to be possible because we lie to them and tell them it is. There will always be a small percentage of us who fluke a drug-free birth in hospitals and if women want this, they should be able to access it. The problem is that a profitable, woman-hating propaganda designed around the false notion that birth itself is intrinsically dangerous, is not going to give women the normal birth they desire for them and their babies without a lot of luck or maybe a lawyer present. So I fervently want those women to be able to decide what happens to them as much as I want the actions of my own body to be solely under my control. And I want all women to know that this is their right as human beings.

Picardie Cadence

I learnt love later in life
It was taught to me via brutality
I learned it from hatred
From raw power which sought
to subjugate me
by people in uniforms with guns
who peered over my naked body
making demands of me
By people who so fear death
they kill to defend themselves against it
From people who sought access to
what they saw as my poison
to use it against me and crow
that I was the killer
and they the champion of my child
Endless showings of the moment
I birthed
on a giant screen
in a crowded courtroom
filled with cameras
all seeking the witch mark on my raw flesh
But sadly for the mob
And the ones with the guns
I was not cowed
and I learnt love

I learnt it to be limitless infinite beyond myself
and within myself
So I can look at their sad collapsed lives
and feel little beyond pity
that we can live with so little connection
to our own humanity
Incapable of extending it beyond
the borders of our own flesh
But I know that love in full flight
is an unaccustomed sight
and I try to keep it contained
hidden under my skin
buried in my long-scorned flesh
If you stray too close
or touch me
I will spark and startle you
Hold fast
It is only love
It is not the snare you were told
to warn you from it and what it brings
And
here's the kicker no one tells you
This is no special feat of mine
This is the mere gift of all humanity

Endnotes

1 "… we are committed to promoting the additive use of gender-neutral language in traditionally woman-centric movements (birth and reproductive justice) …"; <https://mana.org/healthcare-policy/position-statement-on-gender-inclusive-language>
2 <https://www.feministcurrent.com/2015/10/13/are-we-women-or-are-we-incubators-an-interview-with-marylou-singleton/>
3 A hysterotomy is an incision made in the uterus.
4 Sheila Kitzinger, *The New Pregnancy and Childbirth* (London: Dorling Kindersley, 2003/2011, 4th revised edition).
5 <https://www.theguardian.com/australia-news/2018/jun/28/a-decade-after-the-butcher-of-bega-red-flags-continue-to-be-missed>
6 <https://theconversation.com/factcheck-is-suicide-one-of-the-leading-causes-of-maternal-death-in-australia-65336>
7 "For the master's tools will never dismantle the master's house. They may allow us to temporarily beat him at his own game, but they will never enable us to bring about genuine change." Audre Lorde, 'The Master's Tools Will Never Dismantle the Master's House' in *Sister Outsider: Essays and Speeches* (Berkeley, CA: Crossing Press, 1984/2007), pp. 110–114.
8 "Gaye Demanuele and the politics of homebirth" by Petra Bueskens; <http://petrabueskens.com/gaye-demanuele-politics-homebirth/>
9 Feminists in the 1970s were quick to note the connection between witches and healthcare: see the classic book *Witches, Midwives and Nurses: A History of Women Healers* by Barbara Ehrenreich and Deidre English (Old Westbury, New York: Feminist Press, 1973).
10 A brief outline of the relevant inquiries and campaigns can be found here; <https://www.pregnancy.com.au/the-campaign-so-far/>
11 In 2020, Scott Morrison is the Australian Prime Minister.
12 Midwife Lisa Barrett was found not guilty of manslaughter; <https://www.abc.net.au/news/2019-06-04/former-midwife-lisa-barrett-found-not-guilty-of-manslaughter/11173254>
13 <http://harriettehartigan.com/birth-is-as-safe-as-life-gets/>
14 Miranda Devine wrote this article which appeared in *The Daily Telegraph;* <https://www.dailytelegraph.com.au/price-of-belief-may-be-a-babys-life/news-story/32419298d0671a455d188914e9b94afe>

15 'Gaye Demanuele and the politics of homebirth' by Petra Bueskens; <http://petrabueskens.com/gaye-demanuele-politics-homebirth/>

16 Rachel Reed, 'The Future of Midwifery and Homebirth in Australia'; <https://midwifethinking.com/2014/01/02/the-future-of-midwives-and-homebirth-in-australia/>

17 Marjorie Tew, *Safer Childbirth?: A Critical History of Maternity Care* (London: Chapman and Hall, 1990).

18 Marjorie Tew, 'Epilogue: drawing fair conclusions from factual evidence' in *Safer Childbirth?: A Critical History of Maternity Care* (London: Chapman and Hall, 1990), p. 374.

19 ibid.

20 ibid.

21 A term used by Majorie Tew in her book, op. cit., p. 77

22 The Ombudsman's report of reviewable deaths in 2008 and 2009 can be read online; <https://www.ombo.nsw.gov.au/__data/assets/pdf_file/0004/4297/Reveiwable-Child-deaths-2008to2009-Report.pdf>

23 Kevin Fiscella, 'Does prenatal care improve birth outcomes? A critical review' in *Obstetrics & Gynecology* (March 1995) 85(3), pp. 468-79; <https://www.ncbi.nlm.nih.gov/pubmed/7862395>

24 Mika Gissler and Elina Hemminki, 'Amount of antenatal care and infant outcome'. *European Journal of Obstetrics & Gynecology and Reproductive Biology* (July 1994) 56(1), pp. 9–14; <https://www.sciencedirect.com/science/article/abs/pii/0028224394901465>

25 Janet Fraser, interviews for conference paper, Australian Motherhood Initiative for Research and Community Involvement (AMIRCI) conference 2019.

26 ibid.

27 'Government seeks advice on covering stillbirth autopsies in effort to prevent further deaths'; <https://www.abc.net.au/news/2019-07-04/stillbirth-autopsies-government-advice-research/11276286>

28 <https://www.aph.gov.au/Parliamentary_Business/Committees/Senate/Stillbirth_Research_and_Education>

29 Susie O'Brien's article can be found here; <https://www.heraldsun.com.au/news/opinion/home-births-a-major-risk/news-story/5830f3556134634e9786508c221132a1>

30 Mia Freedman's article can be found here; <https://www.mamamia.com.au/freebirthing-her-baby-died-yet-freebirthers-still-want-you-to-try-it/>

31 <https://www.heartfelt.org.au/>

32 To find out more about making placenta prints, see <https://www.verywellfamily.com/how-to-make-a-placenta-print-4111073>

33 My poem 'The Day Before' was first published in *Grieve*, Hunter Writers Centre, 2017.

34 Here is a relevant article: 'Homebirth advocate Janet Fraser lied about long labour, inquest hears'; <https://www.dailytelegraph.com.au/news/nsw/homebirth-advocate-janet-fraser-lied-about-long-labour-inquest-hears/news-story/6c7d2ff170e0f06a51bb21f1ad93f7cb?sv=6430373a5088159ec3fba8fe07f836b9>

35 'Inquiry into Janet Fraser's homebirth finds midwife could have saved baby during delivery'; <https://www.perthnow.com.au/news/inquiry-into-janet-frasers-homebirth-finds-midwife-could-have-saved-baby-during-delivery-ng-caaef13df2fe9fbee9c465c9c1086759>

36 'Women damned if they show emotion, damned if they don't'; <https://www.smh.com.au/politics/federal/women-damned-if-they-show-emotion-damned-if-they-dont-20110211-1aqkw.html>

37 This sad story was discussed in *The Age*; <https://www.theage.com.au/national/victoria/twins-die-in-tragic-hospital-bungle-20111124-1nvjq.html>

38 A hindwater leak is a small hole that opens in the sac up behind the baby's head. Hindwater leaks can continue as a slow dribble, or stop after a while.

39 'Born Free: Unassisted Childbirth in North America', by Rixa Ann Spencer Freeze, PhD thesis, University of Iowa 2008, can be accessed online, see pp. 104–113 for a discussion of 'birth rape', the term first used by Leilah McCracken; <https://ir.uiowa.edu/cgi/viewcontent.cgi?article=1387&context=etd>

40 *The Sydney Morning Herald's* headline on 28 June 2012 can be found here; <https://www.smh.com.au/national/nsw/babys-death-due-to-rash-mother-says-irate-coroner-20120628-215a2.html>

41 'Why was Michael Atkins granted immunity in the case of Matthew Leveson's disappearance?'; <https://www.abc.net.au/news/2016-11-11/matthew-leveson-michael-atkins-immunity-explained/8010190>

42 For evidence of stillbirth rates, see page 5 of the Report from the 2018 Senate Select Committee on Stillbirth Research and Education where it states that "Australia is one of the safest places in the world to give birth, yet six babies are stillborn here every day, making it the most common form of child mortality in Australia"; <https://www.aph.gov.au/Parliamentary_Business/Committees/Senate/Stillbirth_Research_and_Education/Stillbirth>

Other books by Spinifex Press

Karu: Growing Up Gurindji

Violet Wadrill, Biddy Wavehill, Topsy Ngarnjal
and Felicity Meakins

In *Karu*, Gurindji women in the southern Victoria River in the Northern Territory of Australia describe their child-rearing practices. Some have a spiritual basis, while others are highly practical in nature, such as the use of bush medicines. Many Gurindji ways of raising children contrast with non-Indigenous practices because they are deeply embedded in an understanding of country and family connections. This book celebrates children growing up Gurindji and honours those Gurindji mothers, grandmothers, assistant teachers and health workers who dedicate their lives to making that possible.

This book, accompanied by striking photos and artwork, is not only a gift to mothers, but everyone who values children.

—Dr Anita Heiss, Wiradjuri Nation, author and Professor of Communications, University of Queensland

Beautifully written by First Nations women on Gurindji country where the fight for equal wages began. This book passionately expresses the stories told by strong women about their history and culture. A must read!

—Senator Malarndirri McCarthy, Yanyuwa Nation, Senator for the Northern Territory

ISBN 9781925581836

Portrait of the Artist's Mother: Dignity, Creativity and Disability

Fiona Place

A memoir and an examination of the politics of disability. Fiona Place describes the pressure from medical institutions to undergo screening during pregnancy and the traumatic nature and assumptions that a child with Trisomy 21 should not live, even though people with Down syndrome do live rich and productive lives.

How does a mother get from the grieving silence of the birthing room through the horrified comments of other mothers to the applause at gallery openings? A story of courage, love and commitment to the idea that all people, including those who are 'less than perfect', have a right to be welcomed into this increasingly imperfect world.

Fiona Place is one of our great truth-tellers. There is no other writer like her.

—Amanda Lohrey, award-winning fiction writer.

This is the story of a woman who defied the conventional wisdom that a child with Down syndrome is to be avoided at all costs ... Her straight-talking self-portrait, which is also a portrait of her son, Fraser, a gifted artist, exposes the enormous pressure on women to terminate unborn children with detectable disorders.

—Fiona Capp, Fairfax Media, *The Age/The Sydney Morning Herald*

ISBN 9781925581751

Shiatsu Therapy for Pregnancy

Bronwyn Whitlock

Shiatsu is a traditional method of treating illness through stimulating points and meridians with the fingers, thumbs and palms. *Shiatsu Therapy for Pregnancy* is an instructive manual for pregnant women, practitioners, partners, and birthing partners caring for pregnant women. The author provides practical solutions to a host of problems experienced during and after pregnancy. From the antenatal classes to the days and hours just preceding birth, non-intrusive remedies are provided.

With early discharge policies now being the norm, women have to fend for themselves and deal with conditions such as arthralgia, leucorrhoea, pain, fainting, urinary incontinence, constipation, and many more. This handbook describes the foundations for using shiatsu to alleviate the symptoms. For those suffering postnatal depression suggestions for lifestyle are a positive addition to assist women following delivery.

It's refreshing to read about an approach that is positive and empowers women to help their bodies stay healthy and balanced during this time.

—Michelle Wright, Shiatsu Therapist

Shiatsu Therapy for Pregnancy is a book I highly recommend to those practitioners wishing to understand the oriental approach to ante-natal and neo-natal woman.

—Cathie Hunter, Director Shiatsu Australia Educational Services, Diversity

ISBN: 9781875559817

Fear of Food: A Diary of Mothering

Carol Bacchi

An illuminating story of motherhood, *Fear of Food* is Carol Bacchi's account of the first two years of her son's life. She battles his rejection of food, encounters dismissive health professionals, and struggles with sleep deprivation and the uncertainties of doing it alone. Provocative and deeply personal, *Fear of Food* is a compelling read.

Amid the current flurry of public soul-searching about work, family, parental leave and childcare, Carol Bacchi tells the struggles of motherhood from the inside.

—Marion Maddox, Victoria University

It's time to speak truthfully about the realities of parenting. Carol Bacchi's candid and moving account of early motherhood reveals how lonely and harrowing it can be when things don't go as expected. Her endurance, courage and unfailing tenderness will console and encourage mothers everywhere.

—Dr Lisa Hill, Research Fellow, University of Adelaide

Bacchi's account has significant cultural meaning in that it draws attention to the wider culture of oppression and undervaluing of motherhood in contemporary society.

—Sheree Gregory, *Post Graduate Review*

ISBN: 9781876756321

Surrogacy: A Human Rights Violation

Renate Klein

Renate Klein argues that surrogacy can never be ethical, and she details her objections by examining the harms done to all those involved, including to the children born of surrogacy.

My eyes have been opened about an issue that was sadly not much on my radar prior to reading her incisive analysis and discussion of the serious and complex problems involved in surrogacy and its allied industries.

—Dr Victoria Kuttainen, James Cook University

Those uneasy about surrogacy will find their disquiet confirmed by this forceful polemic … As a seasoned activist, Renate Klein knows the power of plain language.

—Fiona Capp, *Sydney Morning Herald*

This small but mighty book is densely packed with an examination of surrogacy and her objections to the "dangerous and exploitative nature of the surrogacy process." She boldly and succinctly exposes the dangers and dilemmas of what she calls the "latest frontier of violence against women."

—Kallie Yeoman, MS, BSN, RN, The Center for Bioethics and Culture Network

Surrogacy: A Human Rights Violation a must-read … Klein allows the voices of surrogacy's many victims to be heard.

—Kate Rose, *Dignity: A Journal on Sexual Exploitation and Violence*

ISBN 9781925581034

If you would like to know more about Spinifex Press, write to us for a free catalogue, visit our website or email us for further information.

Spinifex Press
PO Box 105
Mission Beach QLD 4852
Australia
www.spinifexpress.com.au
women@spinifexpress.com.au